THEY
WALK
ALONE

The Tragic Journey of Dementia

It is pure torture to watch a loved one slowly lose everything and know there is nothing that can be done for them

Chapter 1
The Fall

January 1, 2000, arrived and the world had just survived the Y2K scare without a glitch. No Armageddon. No worldwide computer crash as the year turned from '99 to '00. The scare turned out to be just that: a scare. Just the beginning of another year, like every New Year's Day in the past. Except, this year, I found myself traveling down a fork in the road that would impact me for the rest of my life.

Mamaw was no longer living alone in New Castle because of her dementia. She had moved into my sister Laura's house in Waldron, Indiana. Her dementia had progressed far enough that it wasn't long before she thought she had always lived there. She still remembered her family members. It was obvious, though, that Laura and Mom had made the right choice in moving her out of her own house. She was in no condition to continue living alone and unsupervised. Living with Laura allowed her to fall into a routine each day that was more comforting to her. After all, her whole life had been one of daily routines.

Super Bowl Sunday rolled around on January 30, 2000, and Mom decided to come to Bedford to watch the game with me. She brought Mamaw with her because she knew how much she liked to come and see me whenever she could. I don't remember much of that day, other than the fact that the Saint Louis Rams beat the Tennessee Titans. I've seen enough highlights to know Steve McNair made a valiant attempt to win the game, coming up a mere foot short as the clock ran out. The entire day seems wiped from my memory before the moment when Mom decided it was time to leave.

Everybody said their goodbyes and I remember giving Mom and Mamaw each a hug and kiss before returning to my recliner. The living room was a sunken one, with a two-foot drop from the open hallway and dining area to the living room floor. The front door was next to one end of the drop-off. The steps down into the living room were on the opposite end. This was where the enclosed hallway leading to the bedrooms began.

As they neared the front door, I yelled, "Bye, Mamaw!"

Mamaw turned toward me and said, "Oh my, I forgot to give Bobby a kiss," and she continued to move toward me, oblivious to the two-foot drop-off.

I knew what was going to happen as soon as she turned in my direction. I shouted for her to stop as I jumped up and ran to intercept her, even though I knew I couldn't possibly get to her in time. I watched helplessly as she stepped between the couch and the wall and dropped straight to the floor. Mom jumped down to her side, and I was there a second later. She was so frail I was certain she had seriously hurt herself.

She complained that her leg was hurting badly. Mom checked her out and decided we should take her to the hospital for an X-ray. I picked her up and carried her in a seated position to the van. I couldn't believe how light she was. Mamaw had always been thin, but she must have lost a considerable amount of weight. She was light as a feather.

I drove her and Mom to the emergency room where Mamaw was quickly checked in. The doctor on duty came in and sent her off for an X-ray. Sure enough, just as expected, she had broken her leg. The leg was broken at a point high up the calf and required surgery to set it properly. They put a strap-on cast around her leg and wrapped it with Ace bandages to keep it immobilized through the night. Because Mamaw had to spend the night in the hospital, she was transferred from the emergency room to a private room.

I told Mom I was going to spend the night with her at the hospital. I wanted to make sure she didn't get disoriented or scared during the night. I thought my being in the room with her would make it easier. I could also make sure she didn't try to get out of bed and hurt her leg even more. Mom waited until Mamaw was comfortably settled into her room and had at long last fallen asleep, then went back to my house for the night. I was tired, so I checked on her one more time to make sure she was sleeping all right. Thanks to the pain medicine, she was still sleeping soundly. I kissed her on the forehead before sitting down in what was supposed to pass as a recliner in the hospital room. I thought it was going to be a long night because I couldn't find a comfortable spot in that chair. Trust me, I tried every conceivable position, to no avail.

I was wrong. One minute, I was tossing back and forth, praying that dawn would hurry up and arrive. I was getting more and more frustrated by the moment with the chair. The next thing I knew, I was waking up to the sound of my dear, sweet grandmother giving the nurse an earful. I couldn't believe it. I had never heard her so much as raise her voice at anyone, not even one of us five grandkids, who had certainly tested her patience on many occasions. Yet, there she was, giving it to this poor nurse.

I couldn't quite understand what she was so worked up about, and was worried something was wrong with her leg. I got to her bedside and asked her if she was all right. She proceeded to tell me how she was sound asleep when this woman had come into her room and turned the lights on and awoken her. She continued, telling me how it wasn't right and that they shouldn't be waking people up in the middle of the night. Wow, she was fired up about this! I explained they needed to take her temperature and her blood pressure to make sure she was doing all right. She didn't understand why this was so important and wanted to know why they couldn't let her sleep and do it in the morning. She was really mad.

Then she wanted to know where her panties were.

I must admit, this caught me off guard. Our conversation had just taken a major turn into unchartered waters. This was something I had never, ever expected to be discussing with my grandmother. Or anyone, for that matter.

"What do you mean, where are your panties?"

"I woke up and I didn't have any panties on. Somebody took my panties!"

Then I understood. "Mamaw, you hurt your leg at my house. Do you remember doing that?"

"Well, yes, I think I do remember doing that. Is that why this big old thing is on my leg?"

"Yes, they had to put you in a cast. We're still in the hospital. They had you undress when we got here so you could change into a hospital gown before they X-rayed your leg. Do you remember that?"

"No, not really. Well, why did they make me take off my panties?"

"It's their policy. It's going to be all right, Mamaw."

"Okay, Bobby. I'm sorry. I was just confused. So why do I have this big, heavy thing on my leg?"

"You broke your leg, Mamaw. Do you remember stepping off the edge of my living room and hurting it last night?"

"Yes, I remember." And with an embarrassed smile, she said, "I don't know what's the matter with me."

"It's alright, Mamaw. I'm right here with you and I'll be here all night."

"Okay, sweetie, thank you."

"All right, Mamaw, let's let the nurse check you out so we can turn the lights back off and you can go back to sleep. Is that okay with you?"

"Sure, honey, that's fine."

The nurse went back to checking all Mamaw's vital signs and gave her another dose of pain medicine. I kept talking to Mamaw about trivial things to distract her while she was going through this. I asked if she was cold, and was she thirsty? Could I get her another blanket? Anything to keep her focused on me and not the nurse. I didn't want her attention to wander back to the poor nurse, and I *didn't* want to have another discussion about her panties.

I tucked Mamaw back into the bed and sat by her side until the medicine kicked in and I could hear her snoring. I silently said a prayer that she would sleep through the night as I returned to my oh-so-comfy chair in the corner. I began another round of tossing and turning, once again certain I wasn't going to get any more sleep tonight. The next thing I knew, I was awakened by the lights coming on and the voice of my grandmother, once again, giving the nurse another earful! Uh oh. I hadn't considered the fact they had to check her vital statistics every two hours.

I intervened right away and calmed Mamaw down as best as I could. As much as I had hoped to avoid it, I had to play another round of "Where's my panties?" with her. I calmly talked her through things until I could get her to some point of clarity. She seemed to grasp that she was in the hospital and remembered breaking her leg. She took a little longer to calm down from being woken up this time, probably because the pain medicine was building up in her system and adding to her disorientation.

The biggest issue for her was she couldn't understand why they had to keep waking her up. The question may not have had anything to do with her diminishing capacities. I didn't understand it myself. Why did they have to keep waking her every two hours when they had all those monitors hooked up to her? Was it necessary to have every light in the room on to check her blood pressure, oxygen levels, and other vital signs? Miners can work in an area underground in complete darkness, except for what is emitted from the lights on their helmets. So why does a nurse need 10,000 watts of lighting to care for patients at night? Nurses should wear those miner's helmets on their heads during the night shifts. Or at least carry little pocket flashlights.

I spent the rest of the night jumping up at every noise and checking on Mamaw. If she was awake, I would ask how she was doing and see if she needed anything. I would then have to explain to her once again why her leg was so heavy and remind her of the accident. This went on all night long. As much as I had hoped to avoid it, I'd also have to explain to her each time that nobody had taken her panties. I'd get her calmed down and back to sleep, only to have the lights flipped back on a few hours later and go through the whole routine again. My personal version of the movie *Groundhog Day* went on for the rest of the night. Dawn made its glorious appearance and ended the cycle, and the lights were no longer an issue.

Mom arrived early, so I ran home and showered and went to the hotel. I quickly performed my Monday morning routines and made sure there were no issues from the weekend that needed my attention. When the time for her surgery got close, I returned to the hospital to be with Mom. I went to see Mamaw in the recovery room as soon as she had awakened. When I first saw her in that full leg cast, I couldn't believe how huge it was. It ran from her ankle all the way up to the top of her thigh. That cast looked like it weighed more than she did. Sadly, it did. The leg would have to be non-weight bearing for six to eight weeks to heal, which meant Mamaw was going to need supervision and assistance around the clock.

Mom and I both were friends with Al Estes, the administrator at a nursing home here in Bedford. She met with him about moving Mamaw into his facility for her recovery and rehabilitation. He had a space available, so Mom completed the paperwork to have her admitted for the next few months. Arrangements were made with the hospital to transport Mamaw after her discharge. They took her by ambulance so she would be as comfortable as possible with her leg in the full cast during the move.

7

Mom got Mamaw settled in, and she was an instant hit with all the nurses. Her kind demeanor and the way she talked to everyone like she had known them her whole life made her a clear favorite of the staff. Her dementia was still at a point she could hide it well. The way she referred to everyone as "honey" and "baby" made remembering names unimportant to her. She talked so sweetly to everybody that, for all outward appearances, she was only there to recover from a broken leg. The nursing staff would wheel her out into the hallway so she could people-watch. They were good about speaking to her whenever they went by, and Mamaw, who still loved to talk, could greet people as they passed her doorway.

The surgery seemed to have triggered another effect we would never have predicted. Mamaw forgot she smoked. This wasn't a short-term memory loss. She had smoked for seventy years. But she never asked for another cigarette again, ever. The last cigarette she had was at my house, the day before. It wasn't just the memory that was gone, but the cravings as well. Mom walked with Mamaw past the nursing home's smoking area once. The smell of cigarette smoke tends to linger near designated smoking areas. Mamaw smelled the smoke but had no reaction. No sudden memory of smoking, nothing. She just asked Mom what that room was for, Mom told her she didn't know, and that was the end of it. This always amazed me. At the stage of dementia, she was in when she forgot she smoked, she still had most of her long-term memories. For Mamaw, smoking wasn't just a long-term memory. It was more like a lifelong memory. I remember her telling me she was just twelve the first time she snuck behind their barn and rolled her own cigarette, and she had been smoking ever since.

Mamaw's dementia was still in the initial stages when she fell. She could remember the faces of some of the regular staff that took care of her. This helped keep her from getting disoriented and confused. She also still knew the names of most family members. Living in a full-care facility ensured she got the care she needed, but not the human contact and interaction we all need. It is so important for family and friends to continue being involved in the lives of their loved ones who live in a nursing home. Nurses have jobs and responsibilities, and typically only interact with the resident as their jobs require it. But residents are still people and need to know they are still loved, even if they don't recognize their visitors. Mamaw was eighty-eight years and five months old when she moved into the nursing home.

Chapter 2
Mamaw's Life

Mamaw was born, Thelma Louise Solomon, in Spiceland, Indiana on June 3, 1912. Spiceland is located just south of New Castle on State Road Three. Per the City of Spiceland records, Spiceland was a small Quaker community founded in 1842. During the Civil War era, Spiceland was a major stop on the Underground Railroad used to move former slaves to freedom. This small town is where the franchises for Minute Made Citrus Concentrate and Carnation Evaporated Milk were started. This all happened in a small town with a population of under 900 residents.

Mamaw's parents were William James Solomon (1887-1968) and Mary Ethel Johnson (1891-1956). She was the second oldest of their six children. Her oldest sibling was her sister LuLu Isabelle Solomon (1910-1981). Next was another sister, Agnes Genevieve Solomon, who was born in 1915. George Fredrick Solomon was born in 1920 and Gerald Edgar Solomon was born in 1923. Agnes passed away in 1926 at the age of 11 from a heart condition. Mamaw spoke of how her whole family was gathered around Agnes' bed at the end. She remembers that Agnes kept saying she saw their deceased grandmother before she died. Following Agnes' death, Mamaw's youngest brother, Phillip Everett Solomon, was born in 1928. They were all born in the Spiceland, Dunreith area of Indiana.

All three of her brothers served in the military. Uncle Gerald was in the Army and the Navy during World War II. Uncle George was in the Army during the same war and fought in France. I remember many years ago Marta, Uncle George's daughter, was watching a documentary on famous bridges of World War II. They were showing pictures of these bridges when one came onscreen, and there was her dad, my Uncle George, standing guard with another soldier. My Uncle Phil also served in the military. He was too young for the big war but served in the Navy after it had ended.

Uncle Gerald had taken his family on a vacation to Lake Michigan in 1956. Aunt Donna, his wife, was on the shore with their young kids Kathy, Vicki, Jerry, and Don. Uncle Gerald was a very strong swimmer, so it was not unusual for him to take off swimming towards the deeper water. Aunt Donna recalled later seeing one arm waving before he disappeared. It was a simple gesture and appeared natural for him to be waving at her and the kids. Then he was gone. I can't imagine the panic she must have felt when she couldn't see him anywhere in that vast body of water in front of her. The kids would have been terrified, witnessing their mother's frantic screams for Uncle Gerald. He was thirty-three years old. This was a very tough year for Mamaw and her family because she also lost her mother that year.

Uncle George remained in New Castle his whole life and had always been a huge part of Mamaw's life. His daughter, Marta, resides in New Castle as well, and his son, Bryan, is a retired Nazarene minister who travels the country preaching at Nazarene churches everywhere. Uncle George recently celebrated his ninety-sixth birthday. Uncle Phil moved to Lafayette and was married for many years to my Aunt Nancy, who was taken early in life by cancer. Their kids, Diana and Penny, still live there. Uncle Phil celebrated his eighty-eighth birthday in November 2016.

Mamaw went to high school in Spiceland, Indiana and graduated in 1930. She played on one of the first girls' basketball teams. She also ran track, competing in the hurdles. During her early years, after high school, she had no desire to have children. Then she met Wilbur Louis Davis, my Grandpa Bevo, her soul mate and the love of her life. Mom was born in 1945 and wiped away any sign of the woman who never wanted kids. Mom was the light of Mamaw's life, and she made no secret of it. She didn't have any more children after Mom, convinced she already had the perfect child. Her life revolved around my mom, who was the center of her universe. She was a strict mother when Mom was growing up, but there was never any doubt about how much she loved her. Life was perfect for Mamaw over the next fifteen years, until tragedy struck and Grandpa Bevo passed away in 1960.

Mamaw was devastated. She experienced severe depression from this loss and became overly protective of Mom. She was scared to let Mom out of her sight, even having her sleep in her bed at night to keep her close. Mom wasn't allowed to attend sleepovers with her friends, but she would allow Mom to have friends spend the night. A few years later, in 1962, Mom graduated and married my dad. When Mom left, Mamaw had to snap out of her depression as she was now on her own.

She kept her time filled with a full schedule, but she always found the time to visit with Mom on weekends. I came along on April 16, 1963, and Mamaw became a grandmother. She was no different from any grandparent and came to see her first grandchild every chance she could. On one wall in her living room, she had two large framed pictures of me sitting up in a little suit and tie.

We moved to Indianapolis in early 1964, and my brother Scott was born later that same year on August 4. The first-time Mom told Mamaw she was pregnant, she responded in her typical unfiltered honesty. She said she didn't know how Mom was going to be able to afford another child. She had grown up in a big family of six kids during the Great Depression and remembered how hard it was for her parents raising and feeding so many kids.

Scott was born, and Mamaw was just as crazy about him as she was when I was born. I wouldn't have expected any less from her. Mom found herself having to give Mamaw the news of another baby on the way during the summer of 1965. Of course, she once again had to quietly listen to another lecture on how she wasn't going to be able to afford another child. On February 22, 1966, my sister Laura was born, and Mamaw, in the long run, had a granddaughter. She couldn't have been any happier. Her Sherry Kay had given her three beautiful grandkids in less than three years, and she never once complained to Mom about the number of kids she had. Of course, even as much as she loved Mom and the three new grandkids, it didn't keep her from telling Mom that three was enough.

Like a baseball pitcher on a winning streak, Mom wasn't ready for the bullpen just yet. She found herself facing Mamaw during the spring of 1967 with the exciting news of another child on the way. True to form, Mamaw gave her the speech about how there was no way she could afford all these kids. Life throws its own curveballs sometimes, and Mom had a big one thrown her way during this pregnancy. She would find herself divorced, with three kids, and pregnant. My little brother, James, joined the family on December 4, 1967. I don't know if it was Mom's situation at the time, or if it was because he was such a cute baby, but Mamaw felt a special bond with him immediately. She loved my Mom and each of us grandkids unconditionally, and we knew how much she loved us. But I knew she loved James just a little more – we all did – and it wasn't ever an issue. She referred to him as her "little man" from the moment he was born.

Mom remarried a few years later and would have one more surprise for Mamaw. This time she decided to skip the speech on not being able to afford any more kids. She waited until she couldn't hide her condition anymore before telling Mamaw. My baby sister, Amy, was born on December 19, 1970 bringing the kid count to five in my family. She was a beautiful baby with a head full of the curliest hair. Everybody adored my little sister, and naturally, Mamaw accepted her just like she had the rest of us. Mamaw loved curly hair. I know this because when I was young she was always pushing my hair up when it was wet. She claimed it was making it wavy. I wore my hair longer as a teenager and it was curly and wavy. Mamaw always took credit for making it that way from her playing with it all those years ago. She loved seeing all those natural curls in Amy's hair. As adorable as she was, though, even Amy couldn't take James' place. He would always be Mamaw's little man.

Sesame Street, the Electric Company, and Mr. Rogers' Neighborhood played an influential role in households like mine. The shows came out in the late sixties and early seventies. They were designed to help teach young children from poor families. They turned out to be extremely popular with kids from all walks of life. We all watched this show every morning when we were growing up. We only had four channels back then - the three networks and the Public Broadcasting Station (PBS) which carried these shows. When Amy was little and first learning to speak full sentences, she loved to sing. One of the first songs she learned was the "One of These Things" song from Sesame Street. She always ended the verse with, "Can you tell me fid it is so." Everyone loved hearing this, it was so darned cute, so they were constantly asking her to sing it.

"Amy, sing the 'One of these Things' song."

She'd belt that song out every time like she was performing at Carnegie Hall. She would sing her little heart out at the top of her lungs. She always finished with this final line, "Can you tell me fid it is so." She'd then clap her little hands while we laughed at how cute it was. It didn't matter if she was playing in the dirt or with her dolls. She'd hear, "Amy, sing the 'One of these Things' song." She would

14

continue what she was doing while singing the song like there was no tomorrow.

Mamaw treated us all the same and showed the same amount of love to each of us but James was the only one that she had an endearing nickname for. For a woman who didn't want any children, she was sure full of love for us. She adored her grandchildren and spent as much time as she could with us. I was the oldest, then there was Scotty, Laurie, Mamaw's little man Jamie, and Amy. I never knew for sure why she added the "y", but this was Mamaw, so it didn't matter. Each of us grew up and had our own families and lives and went by Bob, Scott, Laura, James, and Amy. Except with Mamaw. We were always Bobby, Scotty, Laurie, Jamie, and Amy to her until dementia stole her memory of us. I wouldn't have wanted it any other way, and I don't think the others would have either.

In my autobiography of my military career, *We Were Soldiers Too: Serving as a Reagan Soldier During the Cold War,* I shared a story about Mamaw. I was running on base during a morning physical training session with my unit. I ran by my apartment and could see Mamaw sitting on my back patio in her pajamas. She was smoking a cigarette and drinking her morning coffee. I was leading the formation and singing the cadence to keep the formation in step when I spotted her. I waved at her as we passed, motivated by the opportunity to be seen by her. I wanted to make her proud by seeing her oldest grandson leading a formation of army soldiers. I wasn't prepared for what happened next. Seeing me wave, right away, Mamaw jumped up and yelled, "Hey, that's Bobby!" She was waving excitedly back at me while hollering as loud as she could, "Hi, Bobby!" I was the Operations Sergeant, also known as the training noncommissioned officer (NCO), for my company at the time. I worked directly for the company commander and very closely with the company senior leadership. This included the company executive officer, the first sergeant, and all the platoon leaders and platoon sergeants. From that point on, they all referred to me as Bobby. Their little jest reminded me of Mamaw every time they called me that. I'm sure it was done to embarrass me, but it always brought a smile to my face. Thinking of Mamaw has always had that effect on me. I'm sure she had this effect on everyone who had ever met her.

Mamaw worked as a newspaper proofreader for the Courier Times in New Castle, Indiana. She worked Tuesday through Friday from 7 AM until 4 PM, and Saturdays from 7 AM until 2 PM. There were two other women who were also proofreaders. Their job was to read the print proofs for that day's paper and catch every mistake: spelling, grammar, and incorrect sentence and paragraph structure.

Newspapers used to have these huge line casting machines called the Intertype. Each machine had one typesetter who typed the newspaper articles on what looked like a typewriter keyboard. The machine imprinted each word on an aluminum cast. The words were backward and upside down, like a mirror image. Each cast was the size of one newspaper column, about two and a half inches long, and wide enough for one newspaper line. Each one had only a few words printed on them and was about one and a half inches deep. The small diecasts were placed in a box the size of each article. A proof sheet was made by rolling ink on the article and placing the small box in a machine that pressed a piece of paper on it to create the proof sheet. The printed sheet would go to Mamaw or one of the other women to be proofread. They marked any mistakes and returned the proofed sheet to the typesetter. They would look for the small diecast with the mistake in it, pull it out, replace it with a corrected diecast, and return it to the box. Once all the articles were correct, they would be placed in a bigger box the size of one full newspaper page. The boxes for each page were then taken to the print room and inserted into the huge printing press. The press ran enormous rolls of paper across these boxes that were inked and pressed into the paper, over and over, at an extremely fast pace. They then passed through a cutting machine, a folding machine, and a machine that inserted the different sections together. Lastly, they were bundled and tied together to be transported to the paper deliverers' homes. The paper delivery person was responsible for rolling them and slapping a rubber band around each paper.

I remember many times I would spend the night and go to work with her the next morning. Whenever my adventures on my bike took me downtown, I always made sure to stop in and surprise her with a visit. The look of pure joy on her face when she saw me enter the proofreading room made me feel like the most important person in the world. This was one of the things that made her such a special person to me. I'm sure she was just as excited to see my brothers and sisters. She never once seemed irritated or bothered by my unexpected visits. And there were many of them. I always used the backdoor to enter the building, and it opened directly into the diecast room. The whole room was filled with these Intertype typesetting machines that had one person working at each machine. They all knew me and my brothers and sisters by name and always had a kind word for me when I came in. Everyone thought very highly of Mamaw and had a lot of respect for her. She brought joy wherever she went.

She worked for the paper full-time from around 1949 until 1979 when the paper began its transition to a more modern set-up and didn't need proofreaders anymore. She was sixty-seven years old. The paper thought so much of her that they offered her part-time work as the newspaper historian, a position created specifically for her. Her job was to catalog and file all the old newspapers and microfiche film rolls of every newspaper they had ever printed. She cut out stories and articles and filed each away by subject. If someone wanted to research Kent Benson, the famous basketball player from New Castle, they would find the file with his name on it. The file would be filled with everything ever printed about him, neatly cut out of the paper by Mamaw. The time came when the newspaper didn't have any other work for Mamaw and she officially retired.

New Castle continued to be a fanatical town when it came to high school basketball. It was only logical that the state would build the Indiana Basketball Hall of Fame and Museum there. When Mamaw left the newspaper, she volunteered to work at the Hall of Fame. When she first started, she was assigned to the gift shop area. This was perfect for her because it allowed her to visit with everyone who came in. She did this for quite a few years and loved every minute she spent at the museum. Then dementia reared its ugly head and she started struggling with working the cash register. Whoever was in charge when this happened, God bless them. They knew how much Mamaw enjoyed what she was doing. Rather than removing her from the schedule, they moved her to the basketball exhibit. This was an exhibit with an actual goal on a replica of a basketball court free throw area. Mamaw's job was to stand by the foul line and hand visitors a basketball so they could shoot a free throw. This was an awesome decision because it allowed her to continue visiting with people without any technical responsibilities. She continued volunteering a little while longer until dementia forced her to stop a lot of her extracurricular activities outside her home.

One of her favorite things to do when she wasn't working was bowling. She started bowling around 1950 on a Thursday night league at the Rose Bowl on Indiana State Road 3. Many years later, when she got older, she joined a senior league that bowled on Friday nights. She bowled in both leagues well into her seventies, in time, dropping the Thursday night bowling, but stayed in the senior league into her early eighties. I loved spending Thursday nights with her when I was growing up and getting to go to the bowling alley.

She always got to the bowling alley early. We'd sit at the snack bar and eat a hamburger or tenderloin and fries before her bowling league started. She had taught each of us grandkids to bowl at a very early age, so after the two of us ate, she always gave me money to bowl. I'd go to the open lanes at the end of the bowling alley and bowl two or three games by myself. When I finished, I'd go get enough change from her to buy a Yoo-hoo and sit with her and her teammates to watch them bowl. I can remember how proud she always seemed to be when I would come sit with her in the team seats. This made those bowling nights even more special. Truth be told, she was an excellent bowler and I enjoyed watching her bowl. I spent most of my time distracted by the bowling going on in the other lanes. But when it came time for Mamaw to bowl her frame, I was completely focused on her lane. In those moments, I was just as proud to be her grandson, sitting among her teammates, as she was having me there. I am 100 percent sure my mom and each of my brothers and sisters felt the same way at the bowling alley when they were with her. She was an incredible bowler, even in her later years.

She was the secretary-treasurer of the Thursday night bowling league for many, many years. Every Sunday afternoon, she could be found at her kitchen table, typing the team score sheets for the previous week on her old typewriter. She would let me type on it sometimes and I couldn't believe how difficult it was to push a letter down hard enough to show up on the paper. It floored me that my tiny little grandmother could type as fast as she did on that thing. She would finish the score sheets and the next morning, drive out to the bowling alley and hang each sheet in the glass cases by the lockers.

She was an active member in Business and Professional Women (BPW) and attended their meetings on the first Monday of each month. Mom recalls the only time she ever saw Mamaw speechless was the year the BPW recognized her as Woman of the Year. Mamaw had no idea she was being bestowed this honor. They had secretly contacted Mom and Uncle George so they would be at the ceremony when she received the recognition. Mom laughs when she recalls how Mamaw heard her name and sat, frozen in stunned silence.

She may have kept herself very busy during the week, but her weekends were always for her grandkids.

Chapter 3
Dewart Lake

Mamaw had a trailer on Dewart Lake which she and Grandpa Bevo had purchased when my mom was young. In the late 1960's through the mid-1970's, there were no major highways. The trip took three hours from New Castle in Mamaw's red Plymouth Dart. The car had no air conditioning other than that provided when the windows were rolled down. I don't recall ever dreading this trip when it was my turn. The distance and the heat were mild distractions that could never dampen the excitement I always felt going to Dewart Lake. The route remains fresh in my mind even to this day. State Road 3 North took us through Muncie and then Hartford City. We then took State Road 5 from Hartford City through Warren. We always passed a truck stop that was one of the two places Mamaw always stopped to break up the trip and feed us. From here, we continued north on State Road 5 to Huntington where Penguin's Point was, the other place we stopped to eat. State Road 5 took us over the Huntington Dam and continued north through South Whitley, where we took US Highway 30 West. We drove a short distance to near Pierceton, Indiana where we turned north onto State Road 13. The trip got exciting from here as we headed north and entered lake country. This was where I could start looking for signs of each lake as she drove past it.

The Pinkerton's owned the small area on the lake where her trailer was located and called it Pinkerton's Landing. Everyone in my family called it the lakes. We called it that because it was in a part of northern Indiana where there were dozens of small lakes. We drove past many of them on State Road 13 North to get to Dewart Lake. I can still recall the excitement building as the car passed some of these lakes, growing stronger and stronger as I got closer to Dewart Lake. I first would gaze left out the window, searching between the trees for signs of the water and Big Barbee Lake and then Little Barbee Lake. As her car approached North Webster, I stared down each road on the right. My heart would begin racing as I caught glimpses of Lake Webster at the end of each road the car passed. At the edge of town, Mamaw turned left, before coming to the huge amusement park on the right with its rides, putt-putt courses, and rows of trampolines. She drove straight a short distance until the road started winding. At this point, I shifted my eyes back toward the left, looking for signs of Lake Tippecanoe. This road wound its way uphill past countless cottages and homes. The road veered right at the golf course and country club. We then drove a short distance before the road turned sharply to the left. This turn was near a small putt-putt course Mamaw took me to each summer. The next intersection with a stop sign always got me so excited I could no longer sit still. Turning right here put us on the road to Dewart Lake.

The lake was getting close at this point and I always had trouble containing my excitement. My eyes were glued to the right, searching desperately for my first glimpse of Dewart Lake. The view of the lake in the distance got my heart rate up even more, but the sight of the Pinkerton's barn was pure joy. I knew the road to Mamaw's trailer was on the other side of it. The road to Pinkerton's Landing was a gravel road that ran between their old, leaning barn and their home.

Turning right at the barn on a gravel road which took us between two fields of corn. After some time, the road met another gravel road on the left, which we took to get to Mamaw's trailer. A little further was another road that ran along the lake towards Mamaw's trailer but it wasn't in very good condition. Turning left and driving down the road parallel to the cornfield a short distance we came to a point where the road forked. Both directions led the same way because the road made a small loop and connected. We always drove to the left and at once, passed two outhouses. A few feet past this was my Uncle George and Aunt Pauline's trailer facing the road. My entire focus at this point would be on their trailer to make sure they were there. They always arrived on Friday. The weekends were always more special when they were at the lake because that meant I would see my cousin Marta that weekend. She was older than me but always made the weekends even more fun. Hanging out with Marta was priority number one when she was around. When I was young, my cousin Bryan would occasionally come with them, but not often. He was busy in college to become a minister and soon had his own family. The sight of their car meant it was going to be another amazing weekend. They were usually lounging on the front porch and I'd be leaning halfway out the window waving like a fool. Like an idiot, I was worried they wouldn't see me in the only car passing their trailer a mere twenty feet from their porch.

Just past them, the road began its turn to the right. On the left of the road were three trailers. The last trailer in that line was Mamaw's forest green trailer. We were fortunate because she had a trailer that was on the waterfront, sitting perpendicular to the lake. The road made the third turn in its loop behind her trailer and passed the silver bullet-shaped trailer of our neighbors, Jack and Janet Austin. Their trailer was next to us and faced the lake. They had two kids, Trent and Margaret. Janet had muscular dystrophy and was confined to a wheelchair, so I didn't see her often. Jack was a mechanic in the Air Force at Grissom Air Force Base a few miles north of Kokomo, Indiana. Their kids were a little younger than me, but I spent quite a bit of time with them anyway. Age didn't matter at the lakes. I remember how awesome it was when Jack would let Trent and I sleep in the back of his pick-up truck. Only boys could get excited about sleeping in the back of a dirty old truck!

Next to Jack and Janet's trailer was a homemade boat-launching site that was dug down and angled toward the water. Small fishing boats could be launched here, but nothing too large. It served more as a sandbox for us. My brothers and sisters and I loved to dig small trenches down the slopes on the sides of the ramp. We'd use small plastic shovels and spoons to build our imaginary rivers that ended in a deep hole at the bottom. We'd pour bucket after bucket of lake water at the top and watch the water flow like a rough river into our make-believe lakes. We did this dozens of times each summer. At least we did until one week that Mom had taken us to the lakes with Mamaw.

All four of us were digging away, lost in our own little worlds we were creating when one of the other three dug into a yellow jacket wasp's nest. The nest emptied as soon as it was hit and attacked us intruders. I managed to escape without a sting, and James only got tagged by a few. Scott and Laura weren't so lucky and got stung more times than could be counted. Their screams of pain were horrible as we all ran from the wasps to the safety of our trailer. Scott and Laura were in agony and there was nothing Mamaw and Mom could do to ease their pain. They stripped them both down to their skivvies on the front porch to make sure there were no more wasps on them. Both were then loaded into the car and rushed to the hospital to get treated. They recovered just fine, but I don't think we ever played in the boat launch again. I wouldn't even walk through it after the attack.

Beyond the boat ramp was a small open field that had a round table and a light overlooking the lake. Everyone used this table to scale and filet the fish they caught. The small open field had a long bench that sat on concrete blocks facing the lake. Someone had put a sign up naming it the Liar's Bench. This was done as a backhanded joke because this was where the fishermen gathered. They liked to sit on that bench and tell the exaggerated stories of their fishing exploits.

The road forked past the fish cleaning station and near the end of the Liar's Bench. The right fork was the final turn in the loop and headed back towards the outhouses to complete the circle. The left fork continued straight, parallel to the lake until it connected with the main entry road for Pinkerton's Landing. In the center of the loop were three trailers positioned like an I. Across the road from Mamaw was a small, oval travel trailer. In the center of the 'I' was a smaller trailer that was the first one that Mamaw and Grandpa Bevo had bought. The last trailer was the largest of the three, and where Stu and Edith Murray stayed. They were an older couple and Stu was the diehard fisherman of the area. They came every weekend and I think he fished every day.

I fished off the end of the pier Mamaw had in front of her trailer every time I went to the lakes. Sometimes, I'd try Jack's pier next to it or the one by the cleaning station that Uncle George and Stu used for their boats. The larger fish were out in the deeper water, so most of the ones I caught off the piers were small in comparison. As a young boy, I never paid attention to the size, I just knew I had caught a fish. Everything I caught went into the fishing basket unless it was obviously a baby. At the end of the day, I would pull the fish basket out of the water and Mamaw and I would walk over to the cleaning station. She let me descale them with a spoon while she would painstakingly filet every fish in my basket, no matter how small. She taught me how to filet the fish myself, in the long run. It was a very proud moment for me the first time she let me go alone to the cleaning station with my catch.

Jack would sometimes take me out with Trent to go fishing on his pontoon. He taught me how to fish with cane poles, which is easy and a real hoot if the fish are biting. Cane poles were originally made from bamboo canes or stalks. Fishermen would take a bamboo shoot and tie a string to the end of it with a hook for a homemade pole. They are now made commercially from fiberglass but retain the original name. The poles I used were Grandpa Bevo's. The pole consisted of three pieces that were four-foot in length. The bottom pole was the base piece with cork on the bottom to stick the fish hook in when not in use. The opposite end of the base piece was threaded for the middle extension piece. The middle piece was threaded on both sides. The end piece of the cane pole was the narrowest and had the fishing line connected to the end. The line was twelve feet long, the same length as the pole when fully assembled. Bluegill fishing during the day with a cane pole was easy. You set the bobber to the depth the fish were found at. The pole was raised straight up in the air and the line was swung out toward the water. The pole was lowered at the end of the swing, dropping the bait into the water. When the bobber went underwater, all I had to do was lift the end of the pole straight up. The hook would set and the fish was mine.

Jack would take us out at night to fish for crappie, which was my favorite time to fish with cane poles. He would tie a Coleman gas lantern to the corners of one side of the pontoon. The bottom of the lanterns would be tied close to the boat causing the light to shine on the water. The light attracted schools of minnows that the crappie fed on and lured them to the pontoon. Jack would let Trent and I use two cane poles each when we fished, and he usually had three or four in the water. This worked great unless the minnows turned our location into a hot spot. We looked like we were doing a Keystone Cops routine. There we were, two young boys and a grown man lifting different poles up and out of the water. Each pole would have a crappie on them, swinging back and forth. No matter how hard we tried, it was impossible to keep from tangling up lines. We dropped newly baited lines in the water while pulling the other pole out with another fish on it, untangling lines as needed. Jack was always patient with us and would set his poles aside while he helped us untangle.

Mamaw paid $200 a year for her spot and that included electricity and water. I had to walk about 200 feet with our water bucket to a spigot that was tapped into an underground water source. A handle on the side of the pipe was used to pump the water out with. I'd pump that handle up and down with my little arms until the bucket was full. I then had to carry it back to the trailer, trying not to lose too much water before I got back. The bucket was placed in the sink and a tin ladle was placed in it that we used to drink from. I can recall nothing in my life that tasted as good as the water freshly pumped from that well, still cool from its time underground. Drinking it from that tin ladle was like a sweet nectar straight from heaven.

Her rent also covered the use of the men's and women's outhouses. Both were two-seaters for efficiency, although I couldn't imagine sharing time inside one with someone else. I always considered that to be alone time. Using the outhouse was the only not-so-pleasant part of my visits to the lakes. I dreaded those necessary trips. They had to be made though. The trick was to hold my breath before entering it. Run inside, take care of business, and get the heck out before needing more air. I sometimes put off answering nature's call too long if I was in the middle of some adventure. I paid a huge price for those moments. I'd wait until I couldn't put it off any longer. My lungs always ran out of air before my bladder emptied whenever this happened. There was no way I could hold my breath that long for the trips that required sitting down. I was a boy so I still tried. I would hold it until my eyes bugged out. Right before I began seeing stars, I would exhale hard, sending all that old air flying out. Instincts always kicked in at this point. My lungs, deprived so long of air, would automatically take in a huge breath. A huge breath of outhouse air is worse than a normal breath ever would have been. I never learned from this experience. The next time I needed some sit-down time, I would stop at my usual spot. This was a safe distance away so I could work up my courage. Courage was something you needed to take this monster on. When I was psyched and ready, I would once again suck in as much air as I could, confident I could do it this time.

It wasn't only the kids who struggled with visits to the outhouses. I don't recall any of the adults ever bringing reading materials with them when they entered the beast.

26

Mamaw went to Dewart Lake every weekend from Memorial Day to Labor Day, leaving on Saturday after work and returning home on Monday. She would drive to Indianapolis and pick Scott and me up on her way to the lakes. She potty-trained Scott at the lakes. He slept in her queen bed, and I would be on the bottom bunk. She would get up with him a couple of times in the middle of the night to take him to the bathroom. She did this until he could make it through the nights on his own. Mamaw was quite proud of this accomplishment. I'm sure it was a nice help for Mom as well.

We moved from Indianapolis to New Castle when I was in first grade and I started going to the lakes regularly with Mamaw then. By the time I was in third grade, she was taking all four of us older kids with her. We rotated weekends with her little man James and me on one weekend and Scott and Laura the next. She got two weeks of vacation each year, and she always spent those at the lake, splitting these weeks with us as well. Amy was too young for this rotation until I got into middle school. By then, I had started working full-time and couldn't make those weekend trips anymore.

Mom had to work constantly so she stayed home with the three kids that weren't at the lakes. She would sometimes get a full weekend off from work and we'd all make the trip to the lakes with Mamaw. When she eventually had a job that gave her vacation time, we'd all get a full week together as a family. Mamaw joined us on the weekends. It was always so much more fun when all of us kids were together with Mom and Mamaw.

Nothing interfered with my turn to go to the lakes with Mamaw. We all felt this way when it was our turn to go.

Her trailer was old and musty by the time we came along, but it never bothered me. In my mind, that trailer was the best place to be during the summer. In fact, a good whiff of something with that distinct smell instantly overwhelms me with memories of Mamaw and Dewart Lake.

The trailer had a good-sized wooden porch and an awning that could be pulled out to cover it. We had a picnic table that was so old the ends of the boards on the top were a bit rotted. Mamaw had to have Uncle George build a wooden top to cover the table that I varnished every summer. It fit right on top of the original table top making the eating surface like new. It was simple to remove so we could store it in a dry place during the week while we were gone.

That table served as more than simply a place to eat. It had seen more games of Yahtzee, Go Fish, and dice than any picnic table ever built.

One of my fondest memories is of the laughter that always carried across Pinkerton's Landing from Uncle George and Aunt Pauline's trailer. I loved the sound of this during the day and into the night when I was in bed. They would spend the entire day sitting on their front porch talking. Uncle George was always a prankster and would poke fun at whoever was nearby and then laugh his head off. Aunt Pauline was just plain funny. She had the best sense of humor and a deep, resonating laugh. Everybody found time to go visit with the two of them. I could always hear laughter emanating from their porch all day long. Uncle George and Aunt Pauline laughed the loudest, and the sound of them laughing always brought a smile to my face.

Some nights, Mamaw, and Mom if she was there, would put us all to bed and go to Uncle George's trailer to visit or play cards. It seemed to me the laughter was nonstop on those nights, and much louder too. I could hear Uncle George's and Aunt Pauline's distinctive laughs. Mom has a laugh that is easily heard as well. Not so much Mamaw. She had a quiet laugh, so just because I couldn't hear her didn't mean she wasn't laughing. I guarantee she was laughing right along with the rest of them. I'm also certain that most of the laughter had to do with something Mamaw had said or done. I am quite certain that Uncle George was the one responsible for provoking it.

Marta once told me how they used to get the biggest kick out of Mamaw's morning strolls to the outhouse. She would be sitting on the porch with Uncle George and Aunt Pauline. Every morning about the same time, Mamaw would come strolling around the bend and pass their porch. She'd walk by with a roll of toilet paper tucked under one arm and waving at them with the other. They got a good laugh seeing how many different pajama pieces she had on each morning. She either misplaced all the matching pieces she owned or put her pajamas on each night in the dark because she never managed to have matches on. She might have a pink pajama top on with yellow bottoms and a blue housecoat on one day and any number of combinations the next.

I'd wake up early in the morning and eat a quick bowl of cereal or go play while Mamaw cooked us breakfast. I would have an hour to kill after each meal was inhaled. I grew up with a strict one-hour rule after eating before I could get in the water. I don't recall any of us ever complaining about this rule. It was something we all accepted, and I followed it. I knew Mamaw had a younger brother, Uncle Gerald, who had drowned so the rule made perfect sense to us. Mamaw was always the official timekeeper and she never showed any signs of irritation during that long wait. She calmly answered each time one of us asked, "Has it been an hour yet?" God love her, she'd get asked this repeatedly after all three meals. It wasn't uncommon for lots of other kids with their own time to wait to congregate at our picnic table for an hour of games. Mamaw was usually inside the trailer doing dishes or cleaning up while we were preoccupied outside. After meals was the perfect time for her to get any chores out of the way. She liked to sit on the porch and keep an eye on us while we swam.

I would usually swim the entire time between meals. We all did. Every weekend, Marta always found time to take me water skiing at least once. She had taught me to ski around the age of seven, and within a few years, she had me kicking off one ski and using the other one. The best part of skiing at Dewart Lake was when the boat pulled me in front of Mamaw's trailer. I would scour the shoreline until I saw her sitting in her usual spot on the porch, and then I'd wave like a fool until she saw me. When she caught sight of me, she always jumped up and returned my wave just as fervently as I was waving at her. I can't even describe the feeling of pure joy I felt seeing how excited she was to see me skiing by. It didn't matter how many passes by the trailer, or how many times I waved at her, she always waved back with the same amount of excitement.

When I got older, Marta would comment that I should be able to ski barefoot, considering how big my feet were. I always thought it looked cool when someone went by skiing barefoot, with the huge spray of water shooting up both sides of their body, hiding them. Watching and doing were two different things, though. The thought of doing this excited me, but it also terrified me. In the end, Marta convinced me to try it.

When I first learned to ski slalom, she taught me to ski to the side of the boat nearest the shore. This is where I would drop one ski and quickly slide my foot into the remaining ski. Skiing barefoot required staying behind the boat, inside the wake, so all the horsepower of the engine was pulling me when I kicked off the ski. I started off on one ski, and once I was up, she would make a loop back toward our trailer for me to kick off the ski. I placed my free foot barely on the top of the water, lightly skipping across the surface. I slowly started easing my other foot out of the ski boot until my heel was free and only my toes were in the boot. The moment of truth came and I quickly pulled my foot out and placed it in the water. My intent was to lean back for balance while keeping both feet together and in front of me. Skiing barefoot is not as easy as it looks, no matter how large your feet are. I had no sooner kicked off the ski when I found myself flying head over heels across the water, swallowing half the lake before coming to a stop. The effects of a near-death experience wear off quickly with a young boy. By the time Marta had picked up my dropped ski and swung the boat around next to my floating body, I was over the recent scare. With some coaxing from Marta (okay, maybe not so much coaxing, just her asking if I was ready to try again,) I found myself nodding my head yes. She began easing the boat forward, feeding me the rope, and off I went – hoping I wouldn't drown this time. After about the fifth near-death encounter, I decided I liked skiing with at least one ski just fine and ended the barefoot skiing experiment.

In the evenings, we could always find some sort of card game or board game going on at someone's trailer. More times than not, Mamaw would be playing games with us kids instead of the adults. Some nights involved game after game of hide-and-seek and occasionally, Marta would even join in the game.

The best nights were when one of the adults would coordinate a pitch-in dinner and cookout. A large bonfire was built in the boat ramp for roasting hotdogs and marshmallows. My brother Scott accidentally ran across the residual embers of a cookout one time in his bare feet during a game of hide-and-seek. We weren't allowed to run around the area without shoes on, so he was scared to tell Mamaw he had burned his feet. They hurt so badly that night in bed that he kept getting up and sneaking outside to soak them in the lake. Mamaw got up with him at one point and asked him why he was getting up so much. Once she had confronted him, he was forced to fess up and tell her what had happened. She never scolded him at all. She hugged him, then put medicine on his feet, and stayed up with him until he felt better and could go to sleep. That was Mamaw.

The days were nonstop activities. Every day from sunup until around nine at night (the time Mamaw had determined was bedtime) I was doing something, usually in the water. The only time I wasn't allowed to swim was if lightning was spotted. Mamaw would let me swim in the rain, though, which was exciting. She would sit on the porch the entire time it was raining, scanning the sky for any sign of lightning in the distance. If she saw any or heard the rumble of thunder, she would holler, "Bobby, honey, you need to get out of the water now." That's all it took. No argument from me. When Mamaw said it was time to get out, it was time to get out. It was the same when she called me in for the night. By the time I heard Mamaw's call to come home, I had put in a very full day of constant motion. Once I stopped, sleep was quick to come.

The trailer had two doors, but we all used the door closest to the lake where the porch was. It entered the living room and kitchen area. Mamaw had a sofa sleeper against the far wall and a small kitchen table bumped up against the kitchen counter. Beyond the kitchen was a hallway with a set of twin-size bunk beds built into one side and drawers and closets along the left. The hallway ended in the main bedroom that barely had enough room for a queen-size bed and dresser. Between the queen bed and the bunk beds was where the bathroom was supposed to be. Since we had no water, there was no need for fixtures or plumbing, so it served as a closet for our fishing poles. It did have a chamber pot in it, only for emergency use in the middle of the night. It rarely got used because none of us wanted to have to empty and clean it the next morning. If I woke up in the middle of the night, I went outside and snuck behind the trailer.

Sleeping arrangements were simple: Mamaw got the queen bed, I got the top bunk, and James got the bottom. If we were all staying, Mamaw put her little man in bed with her. Scott and Laura got the bunk beds and I slept on the couch. We had no air-conditioning in the trailer. With the hot Indiana summers, and high humidity, it could be miserable inside. I was hardly ever bothered by it, though. I would be so tired by the time my body stopped moving that sleep would quickly carry me away until the next morning and another day of adventure.

One summer, toward the end of the lake season, I talked Mamaw into letting me move her car for her. She had gotten rid of the red Plymouth Dart she had driven for as long as I can remember. It was so old it wasn't red anymore, but light red – almost pink. She replaced it with a white Ford Maverick and would drive that for another twenty years, give or take a year or two. She always parked her car on the other side of the shed to keep it out of the way while we were there. She would back it up close to the trailer when it was time to leave so it could be loaded easier. I was fourteen and thought I was ready for this small driving attempt. It looked easy enough. Mamaw didn't hesitate to give me the keys.

It turned out driving a car wasn't as easy as it looked from the passenger seat. I climbed in and started it up. So far, so good! I put the car in reverse and hit the gas. Gravel went flying everywhere as the car sped toward a nearby tree. I hit the brakes, stopping a few feet before a serious collision with the tree. This nearly ruined any chance of Mamaw having that car as long as she did. I scared myself half to death, put the car in park, and turned it off, still sitting right next to the tree I'd almost hit. On shaky legs, I climbed out and headed towards Mamaw to give her the keys back. I'd had enough driving for the time being. This was when I saw her standing by the trailer. She had both hands held up to her face and her mouth wide open. Her face was white as a sheet. Oh my God! I'd given my Mamaw a heart attack! The color returned to her face as she saw me approaching. She moved in my direction and gave me a huge hug. The first thing she asked was if I was all right. That was Mamaw.

The lake season ended on Labor Day. Everyone who had a trailer at Pinkerton's Landing was usually at the lake on this long holiday weekend. They had to close their trailers up and prepare them to sit empty all winter until the next season. On that Sunday, everyone dragged their picnic tables to the road near the Liar's Bench and lined them up for a pitch-in dinner. Cabinets and refrigerators were emptied of perishables and were used to create dishes for this pitch-in feast. And, of course, more than enough different platters of fish prepared with each person's special recipe.

Most people left that day after the dinner, but a few remained until Monday, like Mamaw, to finish up their work. Mamaw would load us kids in her car and we would head for New Castle, putting the lakes behind us until next year. The ride home was typically quiet. It was a somber moment, knowing I wouldn't be back for a long time. It wasn't very comforting knowing school started the next day, either.

Chapter 4
Growing Up with Mamaw

School always started for me the Tuesday following Labor Day. I grew up in an era when kids could learn everything they needed during a school year that ran from Labor Day to Memorial Day. My generation must have done a lousy job raising their kids. The state of Indiana felt it was their responsibility to make up for our poor parenting by deciding the kids needed to be in the classroom more. To accommodate this, they took away a whole month of their summer vacations.

My time with Mamaw didn't end once school began. Every Sunday, she would pick us kids up and take us to church. Mom went when she could, but she worked so much that she could not go many Sundays. Mom and Mamaw wanted to make sure we grew up with the church as a part of our lives. I attended the Friend's Church on Main Street for most Sundays of the school year, until the summer trips to the lakes began. Mamaw made sure I rarely missed a Sunday, which allowed me to serve as an usher for many years, seating everyone who entered my side of the church. I went to Sunday school and took part in a few Christmas plays over the years. I didn't go any other day of the week, but Mamaw went every Wednesday night for the women's sewing circle. The women sat in a circle facing inward and would work on quilting, crocheting, needlework, or some other sewing project. The sewing was designed to keep their hands busy while they visited and talked about the Bible and their families. I'm sure she talked about us grandkids a lot during those meetings. Lord knows we created plenty of stories for her to share.

The best part of Sundays and going to church with Mamaw was afterward because she always took us out to eat somewhere for lunch. I got to eat at different restaurants that were her favorites like MCL Cafeteria, Long John Silver's, and this little diner-like restaurant inside Grant's Department Store. My first choice was always the L&K Restaurant on the southern edge of town. It had great food, but more importantly to me was that Evel Knievel had eaten there. They had a picture on the wall of him out in front of the restaurant as proof. Evel Knievel was popular for two things when I was growing up. The first was all the enormous jumps he made on his motorcycle. He would jump over cars, buses, and anything else he thought would draw a crowd – especially if it would set a world record. The second thing he was popular for was the jumps he *didn't* make. He wrecked a lot, more times than he successfully made the jumps. He claimed to have broken every bone in his body from all the wrecks he'd had. More likely than not, the missed jumps were the main reason for his popularity, and people only watched him to see if he'd crash. But not me. I always wanted him to make the jumps and set new records. So, eating at L&K was cool to me, and the food was good too.

One evening each week, I would ride my bike to Mamaw's house and mow her grass for her. She had always done it herself until I was old enough and strong enough to push the mower, and then she started letting me do it for her. She had a small yard that didn't take me too long to cut, but it did have a steep slope in the front yard going down to the sidewalk. This was too much for her to be mowing by herself, and it surprised me she could even do it. It was challenging for me the first few summers. When I finished cutting her grass, the two of us would walk a block south down 14th Street to Harold's Hamburgers. She would treat me to the most amazing little hamburgers and French fries. The place wasn't anything fancy. Built like a shack with wooden floors, it only had a few tables and a long counter with bar stools for customers. I always liked to eat at the counter so I could watch Harold grilling the burgers right in front of me.

Indiana is fanatical when it comes to high school basketball, and New Castle was no exception. The New Castle Trojans' home court is the largest high school basketball gymnasium in the country and it has been for my whole life. When I was young and went to their games, fans entered at ground level and had to walk down steps to reach the seats below. There was row after row of seats to the court at the bottom. If Indiana is fanatical, then New Castle residents are insane about their basketball team.

My cousin Marta was on the high school cheer team in the early seventies. The cheer team was made up of high school students who wore matching clothes in the green and white school colors with white gloves. During songs, the band played and the cheer team would perform choreographed hand routines. With their white gloves, all moving in sync, it was an amazing sight to see.

Uncle George and Aunt Pauline became season ticket holders in 1947, long before the famous Fieldhouse was built. They had the tickets when Bryan was in school, and the original Fieldhouse was built in 1961. Uncle George kept his seats and attended every game for over sixty years. This wasn't unusual but common in New Castle. Everyone who had season tickets kept and used them for life. Years later, this became a problem, because fans couldn't get tickets to see the games since nobody was giving up their season tickets. When Indiana superstar Steve Alford was young and on his way to high school, this had to be resolved. The school expanded the Fieldhouse by extending the building upward so more seats could be added. This expansion also ensured their title of "largest high school gymnasium" for years to come.

We couldn't afford season tickets, but I loved the Trojans as much as every other kid in town. Occasionally, I would be given tickets and would walk to the high school Fieldhouse to see them play. Nothing was more exciting to a young basketball player like myself than seeing the great Kent Benson. I loved watching him live on the court, dominating opposing teams that dared to venture into our territory. He was a beast, using his size and an unstoppable force against opposing players. Seeing him live was a rare occurrence, as most games, I would have to listen to on the radio. Whenever I could, I would go to Mamaw's house and listen to the game with her.

Kent Benson would go on to play for Bobby Knight at Indiana University. He was part of the only undefeated season the school ever had, winning the national championship in 1976. He played professional basketball primarily with the Milwaukee Bucks for three seasons and the Detroit Pistons for another seven seasons. Steve Alford would also play for Bobby Knight at Indiana University and win a national championship there in 1987.

I loved spending the night with Mamaw on Friday or Saturday during basketball season. We would sit together at her kitchen table and listen to the high school basketball game on her tiny AM radio above her washer and dryer. She liked to keep score and taught me at an early age how she did it. She would write the names of the starting line-up down one side of a piece of paper before the game started. As she listened to the game, she would annotate points and fouls for each player. A number two was written by their name every time one of them made a basket and a number one for each free throw they made. If they got called for a foul, then an "F" went in their row so she could keep an eye on players who were in foul trouble. If a substitute came into the game off the bench, she added their name to the list and kept track of their performance in that row. I cherished those evenings sitting next to her and listening to those games. We rarely spoke until the game was over because we were following the game so intently, to make sure we scored it properly. The only time we broke this silence was if one of us needed to clarify who had just scored a basket. I also broke our unwritten code of silence whenever Kent scored. I couldn't help letting out an occasional cheer with each basket. I constantly added his numbers in my head to see how many points he had scored after each basket. I would lie across my bed during the game and listen to it in my bedroom if I wasn't at Mamaw's house. I always had a pencil and paper in front of me to keep score, just like she had taught me.

Mamaw always had treats in her house that we couldn't afford to have at home. For example, Mom didn't buy cereal with sugar in it. She told us it was bad for our teeth, but I knew it cost more money. Five kids could have devoured the fancy cereals and it would have cost her a fortune. Mamaw always kept the cereals each of her grandkids liked, which meant she always had five different cereals. I loved King Vitamin and I always knew she would have a box of it in her cabinet for me. She kept a cookie jar on the corner of her cabinet that was always full of cookies. She didn't buy the fancy brand names, but when you're not used to cookies, you're not about to complain about cheap ones. The usual cookies that were found in the jar were chocolate chip, sugar cookies, and gingersnaps. She also bought these windmill-shaped cookies with almond slivers in them that were good.

She enjoyed a glass of Coke every now and then, and she didn't mind sharing it with us kids. Pop was rare at my house. We usually made pitchers of Kool-Aid that we drank every day, so drinking a glass of Coke at Mamaw's house was a real treat for me. She had candy dishes on her kitchen table, the coffee table in her living room, and in her family room. These dishes were always full of individually wrapped Brach's hard candy like butterscotches, red cinnamon balls, and the red-and-white striped peppermint candies. She would remove this candy at Halloween and fill it with candy corn. At Christmas, she filled them with this delicious unwrapped hard candy she bought. It always stuck together, and I'd have to break each piece off before eating it. They were all delicious, but my favorites were the ones filled with jelly.

If I drank too much pop or ate too many cookies when at her house my belly would hurt. She warmed up some milk on her stove and crumbled saltine crackers into it to soothe my stomach. If I fell and scraped a knee, which happened a lot growing up, she had this neat spray that made a clear bandage over the wound to protect it. For every other ailment I had, she whipped out her little bottle of Campho-Phenique. This was her cure for everything.

Mamaw's house was a small, square-shaped house with no hallways. I always went to her back door, which opened into her family room – the largest room in the house. Grandpa Bevo had built it back when Mom was growing up. Once I entered the house, walking straight ahead led to the kitchen. On the opposite end of the kitchen was a large opening to the living room. Turning right led to Mamaw's bedroom and from the far side of her bedroom, another right turn led to her tiny bathroom. Passing through the bathroom was the spare bedroom, and on the opposite side of this room was a doorway that exited back into the family room. There were no doors inside Mamaw's house. The bedrooms and bathroom each had these vinyl accordion-like doors that were pulled across the thresholds for privacy.

Mamaw's house was heated by a floor furnace between the kitchen and the living room. It was located under the house and had a huge four-foot by four-foot vent covering it on the floor. The grill got extremely hot from the flames of the furnace and the heat blowing through it. us We all ran around her house in our bare feet when we spent the night. Each one of us had stepped on that hot grill and burned its lines into our feet at one time or another. I can remember practicing my long jumping techniques by running and jumping over the grill when I needed to cross it. That was way more fun than hugging the wall and stepping around it.

Family was always important to Mamaw. I can remember many times when she would take me with her to go visit her sister, my Aunt Isabelle, while she was still alive. She lived by herself in this little white house in the country. It was in the middle of nowhere, or so it seemed to me in my youth. Aunt Isabelle didn't drive anymore, so Mamaw always made sure to keep in touch with her and visit when she could. It was the same thing with her brother, my Uncle Phil, and his wife, my Aunt Nancy. We always made at least one trip to Lafayette with Mamaw to visit them and my cousins, Diana and Penny. They lived about two hours west of New Castle, so the visits were usually shorter than the travel time. This didn't matter to me. I loved those visits. Sometimes, I talked Mamaw into letting me spend a few nights, and Uncle Phil and Aunt Nancy would bring me home. They were also good about driving to New Castle to see Mamaw at least once a year. Uncle George and Aunt Pauline lived in New Castle, so I got to see them quite a bit, which was nice because Marta lived with them. She was their daughter, after all.

We went to two different family reunions every year. Mom almost always went to these. When she couldn't, Mamaw loaded all five of us into her Plymouth Dart or her Ford Maverick and took us with her. The first one was in the summer and was the Johnson family reunion in Lewisville, about thirty minutes from New Castle. Christopher Johnson was my great-great-grandfather on Mamaw's side of the family. He was the father of Mamaw's mother, Mary Johnson. This reunion was a blast because Mamaw's dad was a Solomon. This meant I would get to see Uncle Phil and Aunt Nancy, and Uncle George and Aunt Pauline. More importantly, this meant all my awesome cousins would be there too. If I was lucky, Marta's brother Bryan would surprise us and show up. The other reunion was in the fall and was the Parker family reunion, held in Farmland, an hour east of New Castle. This was Grandpa Bevo's side of the family. His mother was Virginia Ethel Parker. Mamaw never missed this reunion, and I suspect she went to everyone after he passed away. The cool thing about this reunion was we always played a game of softball after the meal, and the adults let us kids take part.

Life seemed to pull me away from Mamaw when it took me from New Castle to Yorktown. Mom had remarried, and we all moved into her new husband's house. After that, it seemed like I only saw Mamaw for certain holidays, or when she came to spend a weekend with us. We moved to Yorktown halfway through my eighth-grade year of school and I didn't see her nearly as much as I used to.

I got my first job de-tasseling corn that next summer, and my trips to the lakes ended. The summer after my freshman year, I was hired as a stock boy at Ross Food Mart, the only grocery store in Yorktown. My good friend Kent Ross worked there as the other stock boy and got me the job. He had a little pull with the owners to get me hired; his dad and uncle owned the store.

Mom and the family went to Tennessee for Thanksgiving in 1978 to be with her new husband's family. I couldn't go because of work, so I stayed home alone while they made the trip. Mamaw drove to Yorktown on Thanksgiving Day and picked me up. We went to a restaurant in Muncie and celebrated Thanksgiving together. As was typical, growing up in my family, if Mom couldn't be with us, Mamaw always was. We had a wonderful time that Thanksgiving with only the two of us.

During my third summer in Yorktown, I moved to Alexandria, Indiana so Mom could be closer to her work. This was another short distance move for us, as it was a 25-minute drive northwest. I went to Alexandria Monroe High School for my junior year. I graduated after just that one year, and joined the Army. I spent close to eight years in the military as an infantry soldier.

Thanks to my mom, no matter where I was stationed in the military, Mamaw always came to see me. She flew her to Germany with my Aunt Francis, who was Mamaw's sister-in-law. Aunt Francis' husband was my Uncle Bob, whom I was named after. Both were widowers, and it was around this time that they became close again. They got together occasionally after church for meals and became travel buddies, at times, to come see me. They spent a few weeks in Frankfurt with my cousin Pat, one of Aunt Francis' daughters. I rode a train to Frankfurt every free moment I had to see Mamaw.

At Fort Knox, from 1983 to 1985, Mamaw made many trips in her car to visit me. I remember one time during the summer of 1984, she drove down to visit me and see my daughter Amber and my newborn twins, Bobby and Robby. She had Aunt Francis with her on this trip and was still driving her white Ford Maverick. I was driving in downtown Radcliff, just outside Fort Knox, when I spotted her going down the highway in the opposite direction. Without considering the consequences, I made the mistake of hollering out my window, "Hey, Mamaw!" and waving, just like when I passed her on my water skis at Dewart Lake. She recognized my voice and forthwith stopped her car. So, there she was, my beloved Mamaw, sitting at a dead stop on a state highway in Kentucky, with her head leaning out her car window, looking for me.

What had I done?

Terrified that she would be in an accident, I did a quick U-turn. I kept my eyes on her the whole time, waiting for the sound of someone slamming on the brakes before hitting her. Fortunately, when I got the car turned around, she gave up the search for her grandson and started back on her way to my house. I was scared to death she would see me in her rear-view mirror and stop again, so I remained a safe distance behind her. We both made it safely to my house.

I was stationed at Schofield Barracks in Hawaii from 1985 to 1988. Mom flew Mamaw to Hawaii to stay with me for a full month on two consecutive summers. Aunt Francis came with her the first summer, and James and Amy came for the second one. I left the service and moved to Bedford, Indiana where work and life managed to give me poor excuses for not going to see her more often. I took on the responsibilities of running two hotels for twelve years, working 70-hour weeks while managing to attend every one of our kids' sports and school events. I was a workaholic who temporarily lost sight of everything outside the boundaries of work and my immediate family in Bedford. I only saw most of my siblings at Mom's annual Christmas party for many years, because of my misguided priorities back then.

I saw Mom at least every month or two. I would take my family and drive to her home in Shelbyville and spend a weekend with her. During the summer months, I might see Mamaw occasionally because Mom was always having her over. Otherwise, my whole life was in Bedford after getting out of the Army. I worked way more than I should have, and what little time I wasn't working was spent at home with my wife and kids. Even though I had misguided priorities, they weren't so messed up that I neglected my immediate family.

Chapter 5
Family Vacations

Mom decided to start having a family vacation so that we could get our whole extended family together for one week a year. This was a wonderful idea because my family always had an exciting time when we got together, with lots of laughing. Mom got the idea while visiting me one weekend in 1993. I had found a place called Patoka Lake Village, near Patoka Lake, which had recently opened for business. They had brand new log cabins and I rented a cabin a several times to get away with my family. Marsha and I decided to ask Mom down to spend a long weekend with us in one of the cabins without our kids. She loved the cabins and the location, and the idea of the family vacation was born. I made every one of these vacations a priority in my life and scheduled my work around them. My family and I never missed any. Every year, Marsha and I, along with our daughter, Amber, and our twin boys, Bobby and Robby, would load the van and head to whatever destination Mom had picked. The first of these vacations was during the summer of 1994. We rented six cabins for all five of us kids and our entire families. Mamaw came to every family function, including these vacations, and Mom always invited Aunt Francis. I had a speedboat docked on a buoy at the lake, so we spent most days on the lake skiing, tubing, and fishing. The evenings found us all back at the cabins for cookouts and pitch-in dinners. And, of course, we played lots of different games with Mamaw, Mom, and anyone else interested in playing. Mom scheduled a short road trip from the cabins for one entire day to the amusement park at Holiday World in Santa Claus, Indiana. The vacation was a huge success, so we came back the next year.

Mom decided to try somewhere new the third year of the annual family vacation, and we went to a state park near Liberty, Indiana on Brookville Reservoir. We rented A-frames and small cabins for the week. The state park had a huge skunk problem. I guess it wasn't so much a problem as an annoyance. The skunks had become desensitized to people and had no fear of us. That was a good thing because they only spray their nasty scent when they're scared. We didn't know they were accustomed to people, though, so it was nerve-racking the first few nights. Evenings of this summer found us all sitting in lawn chairs in a central location and visiting. After sunset, the skunks appeared out of nowhere. It was a gang of twenty or thirty of them! They'd roam right up to us, even walking under our lawn chairs, looking for food. Everywhere I looked, I could see the white streaks that ran down each skunk's backs. They were everywhere. All I could think about was if one of them got spooked every one of them would panic and I would die of a skunk overdose. We realized about halfway through the vacation it would not be so easy to spook them and we ignored them as they had been ignoring us. Not really, as it's impossible to ignore the sight of so many skunks running around. I guess we became desensitized to them.

Mom had bought squirt guns that had water tanks connected to the guns. The cool thing was that the squirt guns squirted a strong stream of water when activated by sound. They came with a headset connected to them with a microphone. The sound of the shooter's voice sent a stream of water squirting out the gun towards the intended target. This was a hit with the adults, all of whom were Mamaw's grandkids. She sat a safe distance back and laughed while we ran around like fools, shouting into those microphones. Being the smartest of the kids, as all first-borns are (though I'm sure the others would disagree with this,) I realized if I sang into the microphone the water would squirt out nonstop. I chased every member of my family around, singing every silly song I could remember. Poor Mamaw would back up anytime I got near her, so I tried not to chase anybody her way. I could tell she loved the spectacle unfolding in front of her. For my grand finale, I filled my water tank and put my sights on my dear mother. Call me crazy, but it was her idea to bring the silly squirt guns. And besides, it was her birthday to boot. I chased my mother all around the cabins singing "Happy Birthday to You" in my best Marilyn Monroe impression. This had everyone laughing hysterically by the end of the song.

Mamaw was still bowling on her Friday night seniors' league. A few years earlier, she had talked Uncle George into bowling on the team with her. I can just imagine how much laughing went on at the Rose Bowl every Friday night with those two there. I'm not sure when exactly she got him to start bowling with her. It does my heart good to know the two of them got so much quality

44

time together through bowling. It was during the winter bowling season of 1996-1997 that Mamaw collapsed at the bowling alley. She was rushed to the hospital where she recovered quickly and showed no side effects from the incident. Her doctor ran all kinds of tests but couldn't find anything seriously wrong that would have caused her to collapse. Mamaw decided to quit bowling as a precaution, but she didn't feel any different and went back to her life like nothing had happened.

Summer rolled around with no more incidents as the family vacation time came. We spread our wings for the fourth year and rented cabins way up north near Lake Erie. This was my favorite of all the vacations. I love to fish and went walleye fishing on a charter boat when I first got there with all my brothers and brothers-in-law. We didn't get to stay out long because they got seasick, and most of our crew was leaning over the side of the boat puking too. After that, I went three times on the walk-on head boats, twice by myself and once with Amy's husband, Aaron.

The main reason this was my favorite family vacation was the games. We played card games like Gin Rummy, Euchre (A card game like Spades) and Spoon every moment at the cabins. Spoons was a card game where everyone was dealt four cards. Teaspoons were set in the middle of the table, one less than the number of players. The dealer would deal four cards to everyone to start the game. They would then draw one card at a time and look at it. They would either keep it and discard one card to the right face down or pass it to the right. The goal is to pick the right card and get all four matching cards such as all four kings. Whoever got all four matched would grab a spoon which sent everyone scrambling to grab one of the remaining spoons. The person who ended up without a spoon lost and had to leave the game. A spoon was removed from the table and more rounds were played, removing a person and a spoon until only two people were left. The person holding the last spoon would win the game. Games are a hoot with my family, especially when Mamaw was involved in them. She had a way of making everything more fun. She'd pop off with whatever was on her mind, unfiltered, and have us all in stitches. She'd talk nonstop and but became distracted often and with ease, so someone always had to tell her when it was her turn. She had this uncanny way of being in left field the whole game. Then, out of nowhere, she'd make a play and say,

"Oh my, I think I just won," or something to that effect, and we would all bust out laughing.

The cabins we had rented were of assorted sizes and shapes. They ran in two rows with a large open area in between them. It was during this vacation that Mom first realized there might be something wrong with Mamaw. She would see Mamaw walking around the open area with a lost look on her face. Sometimes, she saw her standing in one spot looking back and forth before making her way to her cabin. She soon realized that Mamaw was getting confused and forgetting where her cabin was. This didn't happen often. It did happen frequently enough for Mom to know something unusual was going on. She soon realized she needed to keep a closer eye on Mamaw. I don't recall Mom mentioning any of this to me at that time.

The fifth year, 1998, was the last year of these family vacations, and it was back at Brookville Reservoir. This time, we only rented a few cabins because some of the families wanted to sleep in tents. For this vacation, we went to King's Island for a day and spent another day at Medora, Indiana – famous for having one of the banks John Dillinger had robbed. The rest of the week was spent hanging out at the cabins, playing games. Mamaw was always with somebody, and I don't recall noticing anything unusual in her behavior. But I had no idea that Mamaw had begun showing signs of dementia until sometime after that last family vacation.

The earliest signs were very subtle and went unnoticed for a short time. That's the way dementia is, stealing a few short-term memories, or occasional bouts of disorientation, or struggling to remember a word. These incidents slowly increase over time until they can't be missed or denied. Since dementia typically strikes older people, it is regarded as a part of getting old and simply dismissed. This was not the case with Mamaw. Mom knew right away something was wrong with her at Lake Erie in July 1997.

46

Chapter 6
Vascular Dementia

It became obvious to Mom in 1997 that there was more than forgetfulness going on with Mamaw. She began to worry about her driving. It can be difficult convincing someone they are having memory problems, someone who has been so independent their whole life, above all. While she was concerned about how she would get Mamaw to understand the necessity of giving up driving, ultimately Mamaw made the decision for her. She called Mom one day and said, "Sherry, I don't think I want to drive anymore," and she never did. Mom figured she must have gotten lost, and it scared her when she couldn't find her way home. It was also difficult for her to take care of the simple things with her car when her gas station closed. They had taken care of her for many, many years. All she had to do was pull up to the gas pump. The station would pump her gas and check her oil and tires. They always let her know if it was time to schedule any services on her car. Once they closed, it certainly must have seemed overwhelming to her. Mom was worried Mamaw might forget she didn't want to drive anymore and get into an accident. So, she called Laura, who forthright went to Mamaw's house and took her car away.

Mom would visit and see cigarettes in different ashtrays that had been lit and burned down on their own, unsmoked. Mamaw would light a cigarette, set it in the ashtray, and go do something – forgetting she had left the cigarette behind. She'd then light up another one in a different room without a second thought. The scariest part of this happened when she couldn't find her lighter one day. She rolled up a paper towel and caught it on fire using her stove's gas burners to light her cigarette. She then forgot how to turn the burner off, and had to get a neighbor to come over and help her.

Mom bought a home on Cordry Lake and moved into it in July 1998. Concerned with Mamaw's declining memory, she had her come stay with her for long stretches for the remaining part of the summer and that fall. She would take her back to her home in New Castle for a few weeks and bring her back to the lake house for another stay. Mom was deliberately stretching those visits out longer and longer, intending to move Mamaw into her house permanently.

Unfortunately, the best-laid plans don't always get to happen. Right before the time came to move Mamaw in, Mom had a wall in her lower level collapse and nearly destroy her home. Serious work needed to be done to repair the damage and save her home, so the move had to wait. Scott was in Atlanta and I was in Bedford, so Mom, Laura, James, his wife Lisa, Amy, and her husband Aaron took on the tasks of checking on Mamaw regularly.

Mamaw informed Mom in September that she was going to quit bowling. She was too weak to pick the ball up and roll it down the lane. This news was tough for Mom, as bowling had been a part of Mamaw's life since Mom was a little girl. The decision to give it up hit Mom hard. It had to have been a very difficult decision for Mamaw to make.

We had a tradition each year of celebrating Christmas with Mom on the first Saturday after Thanksgiving. Amy had moved into an apartment complex in Greenwood that had a community room large enough for the Kern clan to all gather in. The family Christmas gathering in 1998 was a wonderful time for everyone. They were every year. This one was a particularly great one for Mamaw. She seemed like her normal self and basked in all the attention she received from everyone. Mom drove her back to New Castle that evening.

Sometime in Mamaw's eighties, she had bought a microwave and quit cooking altogether. Mom told her the family was going to start helping with her grocery shopping and asked her what she liked to eat. Mamaw told her about anything if it could be microwaved. Amy made it part of her weekly schedule to shop for groceries for Mamaw and bought already-prepared microwavable single meals. She always brought one or more of her kids with her so they could see Mamaw. Every time Amy showed up, for some reason, Mamaw always seemed worried that she was coming to leave her kids with her to babysit. Amy would laugh at this and explain to her that they were going to take her out to McDonald's for lunch. Mamaw liked going there and getting a hamburger and a cup of coffee. James' wife Lisa would also come every week and would leave her with easy meals she had made at home. She froze them in single portions that needed to be zapped in the microwave. They both spent time visiting with Mamaw and coercing her into eating something while they were visiting.

This worked for a while, but after a bit, Mamaw stopped eating again. Mom contacted a company called Meals on Wheels and paid them to deliver two meals a day to Mamaw's house. Volunteers would deliver a hot meal every day at lunchtime and leave her another boxed meal to microwave for supper. Mamaw liked these meals, and this arrangement worked for quite some time.

One day, Mom went to visit Mamaw and asked her to get ready to go out to eat. When she was ready, Mom was surprised to see the condition of the clothes Mamaw was wearing. Her entire outfit was wrinkled and had quite a few stains on them. They had obviously not been washed in some time. Mamaw had always been an impeccable dresser when it came to going out in public. She would never be seen in a dirty outfit, especially one that hadn't been ironed. Mom would get her cleaned up and into clean clothes then take her to Bob Evans for breakfast. It was during one of these breakfasts that Mom realized how much weight Mamaw had lost. She had always been thin, so losing weight had made her nothing but skin and bones. Her rings were barely staying on her fingers, so loose they could have slipped right off.

Mamaw wore two rings. On one hand, she had a birthstone ring, with the stones for Mom and all five of us grandkids mounted on it. She had lost the original one up at the lakes, doing dishes. I still remember how crushed she was when she realized she couldn't find it. We looked everywhere for that ring, even in the lake. The consensus was it had fallen into the dishpan and accidentally gotten thrown into the lake when Mamaw threw out the dishwater. When I got out of the service and moved to Bedford, I had a new ring made and gave it to her for Christmas. The other ring was one she had had made with the diamonds from the wedding ring that Grandpa Bevo had bought her. Sitting with her at Bob Evans, Mom couldn't believe how loosely the rings rested on Mamaw's fingers. They talked about this, and Mamaw surprised her by removing her birthstone ring and handing it to her. She told Mom that she wanted her to keep the ring before it got lost.

Mom scheduled a visit for Mamaw with her doctor to check on the drop-in weight and memory loss. He ran some tests and found some brain atrophy, confirming dementia as the cause of the memory loss. It was only going to get worse as it continued its dreadful assault on her brain. Without any warning signs, Mamaw took off her remaining ring while they were at the doctor's office. She handed it to Mom and curtly told her she might as well have that ring since she had already taken the other one from her. It's very common for dementia patients to become depressed when they start forgetting things. Doctors typically put them on an antidepressant. Her doctor decided to put her on one that day as a precautionary measure, even though she showed no signs of being depressed.

The anti-depressant, unfortunately, caused Mamaw to lose her appetite, and so the delivered meals began piling up. When different family members stopped by to check on her, they found that few of her meals were touched. She became sleepy from inactivity and before long, Mamaw started sleeping most of the day. It got so bad that she stayed in her pajamas all day. This didn't go on very long, as Mom didn't hesitate to take her off the medicine. Sure enough, Mamaw started eating again and returned to a fairly alert state of mind.

She didn't experience a full recovery, however. Dementia doesn't work like that. But once the antidepressants were stopped, she could carry on conversations and regain some of her appetite. She was still slowly losing her memory, and there wasn't anything earthly that was going to change this. Mamaw called Mom one day, telling her she needed her help. When asked what was wrong, she said she couldn't remember how to write out a check. Mom told her not to worry and that she would be on her way over soon to help her. Mamaw called her three times within half an hour that day with the same problem. She had not only forgot how to fill out a check, but she had also forgotten she had already called her daughter for help. Such a terrible disease.

November 1999 rolled around and we came to Amy's for another Christmas gathering. Mamaw was noticeably different from the previous year's celebration. She was more withdrawn and spent most of the party pacing the floor. Laura volunteered to drive her home once the Christmas party was over. On their way to New Castle, Laura impulsively asked Mamaw if she'd like to go home with her for a while. Mamaw shocked her by responding that she would like to do that. Laura was ecstatic with her response and drove straight to her home in Waldron, Indiana before Mamaw changed her mind.

Laura's only concern about this arrangement was her dog. She had a huge Rottweiler that didn't know she was a dog and was significantly larger than Mamaw. The dog ran around that house like she was a little kid, always jumping on everyone for attention. Laura was scared to death the dog would tackle Mamaw in search of affection and hurt her. Shoot, she was so big a simple bumping into Mamaw would have been catastrophic. But dogs are smart, even smarter than given credit. Laura's dog must have sensed something about how fragile Mamaw was because she always moved gingerly in Mamaw's presence.

After about a week, Laura said, "Mamaw, don't you think we should go and get you some more clothes from your home?"

Mamaw agreed and they drove to New Castle. When they walked into her house, Mamaw looked at Laura and asked, "You're not going to leave me here, are you?"

Laura's eyes filled with tears and she grabbed Mamaw to give her a hug.

"No, Mamaw, I'm not going to leave you here."

Laura gathered as many clothes as she thought Mamaw would need, and they headed back to her house in Waldron. Moving Mamaw into Laura's house seemed to work very well. She never asked about her home in New Castle and acted like she had lived with Laura her whole life. She didn't spend a lot of time by herself now that she was at Laura's, either. There was always someone for her to talk to and to make sure she ate. Laura and her kids all took the task to heart, and Mamaw couldn't have been in better hands. They took great care of her, and the issue of Mamaw's dementia seemed to be solved for the moment.

Then came that fateful trip to my house and her fall. As tragic as this was – and without sounding too morbid – it was a blessing to me. Having Mamaw in Bedford gave me a chance to make amends for all those years of not spending as much time with her as I should have.

When Laura came to visit Mamaw for the first time following the accident, with that beautiful smile of hers, she said, "I trusted you to take care of Mamaw for one day, that's all you had to do. She never got hurt at my house."

Whenever Laura visited Mamaw in Bedford, she always made sure to remind me of this.

After Mamaw's fall, I reserved a room at Stonehenge Lodge and Mom moved into it the same day Mamaw moved into the nursing home. She planned to stay in town for the first week, longer if necessary, to make sure Mamaw transitioned into the nursing home without any problems. She thought staying in town would be easier for her to be with Mamaw than having to drive all the way out in the country to my house.

Mom found Mamaw a local doctor to be her care provider while she was at the nursing home. He ran some basic tests to discover more about her dementia. He told us the form of dementia Mamaw had was vascular dementia. He believed that when she collapsed at the bowling alley she'd had a mild stroke. A stroke would have cut off blood flow to her brain for a very short period of time and killed some of the brain cells. Since it was a mini stroke, the damaged cells must not have been significant enough to have shown up on any tests her doctor in New Castle ran. This explains why so many years had passed before the symptoms became noticeable.

The Alzheimer's Association reports vascular dementia is the second leading cause of dementia; Alzheimer's is the most common. Like most illnesses, early diagnoses can allow the use of certain medicines to prolong the unavoidable, by slowing down some of the early symptoms. Unfortunately, these two causes of dementia can't be cured. Both conditions are overlooked because they typically hit older folks first. Society tends to consider memory loss as a normal part of getting old. Think about how many times you've heard someone say, "Keep an eye on grandpa, he's getting senile in his old age." This misconception allows dementia to progress further along before it's noticed. By then, the mental decline has already reached a point where it can't be slowed.

I tried to visit Mamaw every day after she moved into the nursing home. She was in a wheelchair during the day so that her leg could be kept straight out in front of her. She was too weak to push herself around, although she could scoot just a little, but nothing significant. She spent most of the day in her wheelchair, which was a far sight better than spending it in bed. The nurses were good about getting her up in the morning, dressing her, and setting her in her wheelchair where she would remain all day. They would push her to the dining rooms for her meals, and to the activity room for special events, and church services on Sundays.

Mamaw's roommate's name was Mary. She was a sweet woman who wasn't a conversation starter, but she was a good listener. This made her the perfect roommate because Mamaw loved to talk. It was very reassuring knowing she was going to keep an eye on Mamaw and could help her when she got confused.

The nursing home was huge and the hallways ran in the shape of squares with rooms on each side. The whole layout formed two adjoining squares, with courtyards in the center of each. The first courtyard was designed for the view from the patient's rooms and the residence couldn't access it. The second courtyard had a sliding glass door found in the center hallway, which opened to a covered concrete patio. The nursing home had rabbits running loose inside this courtyard.

When I entered the main entrance of the nursing home, I went past the administration office and continued straight down the hallway to Mamaw's room. She was in room 112 on the left side of the hallway. At the end of her hallway and to the left were the full-care patients who needed help with everything. Like all dementia patients, Mamaw would, in due course, end up here. Traveling down the hallway to the right were more rooms on each side before ending in the main dining room where most of the residents ate.

I liked to bring my young granddaughters with me on the weekends to visit Mamaw. My wife and I both wanted to make sure they got to know their Mamaw. She still dearly loved kids and was always excited when the girls came with me. She always asked where the girls were when I showed up without them. Sage was seventeen months old and was walking well when Mamaw fell at our house. Jade was only three months old when it happened, so she traveled by the Papaw-powered stroller for our visits the first few months of the year. The girls ended up bringing joy to many of the residents.

There's a reason older family members don't want to end up in a nursing home. For a while, nursing homes had a bad reputation, and rightfully so. Unfortunately, the industry had many unscrupulous operators in the seventies. They provided as little care as possible to their residents, which was outright negligence. By the eighties, regulations were set in place that included regular inspections, which cleaned up the industry. But the real reason many older people don't want to end up living in a nursing home is neglect by their own families. They don't want to be dumped in one and then be forgotten.

I could see the truth of this because I visited Mamaw every day. I rarely saw any other family members visiting other residents during the week. Granted, I was only at the facility once a day, sometimes twice, but my visits were at random times. They depended on when I could get away from work to spend an hour or more with her. I would see a few visitors on Saturdays, but I am confident these were family members from out of town. That's when Mamaw got visits from members of our amazing extended family, so it made sense that this would be true for the other residents. I could see that Sunday was when there were the most visitors. Many families would stop by the nursing home to visit their loved ones after church. I assume this was the most convenient time for them, and it was the one time they had the whole family together. I am not discouraging this because at least they visited. The problem is that this meant the residents didn't have any contact with family members or people who loved them during the week. The only interaction they got the rest of the time was with caregivers and other residents. I did see many preachers and other church representatives stop by on Sundays to administer communion to members of their church that were now residents. But Sunday nights were like the rest of the week, very few visitors.

I think this confirmed my belief that older folks are afraid of being forgotten if they get put in a nursing home. Many the residents in Mamaw's section retained their mental capacities and could carry on a conversation, so I made a point of always greeting them when I passed them. I got to know quite a few of them throughout the facility over the years. I always tried to spare a few moments to speak with them whenever I saw them. I could tell how lonely they were by the way they lit up each time I stopped to talk to them. They were genuinely glad to see me, which was rewarding to me as well. My two little granddaughters were always a huge hit with the residents when they were with me. They all loved seeing Sage running up and down the halls, and her laughter brought smiles to everyone. During that first year, when other residents saw me pushing the stroller with Jade in it, some would wave me over to get a better look at her. Most of them would impulsively reach down and lightly stroke her cheek, commenting on how pretty she was. Seeing and having contact with a baby always made them grin from ear-to-ear. This made me happy too. Bringing the kids along turned into something much bigger than simply letting them get to know their Mamaw. They were too young to remember any of their visits and all the happiness they spread around that nursing home, but I certainly do. They vaguely remember Mamaw but they do remember the rabbits.

The winter months were too cold to take Mamaw outside. I always wanted to get her out of her room when I visited to give her a change of scenery. I would take her down the hallway to the right from her room, toward the administrative area, and then turn left. This hallway opened into a visiting area with couches and chairs on one side of the hallway and a four-seat table on the right that was next to windows. I liked to bring her to this spot so she could look out the window while we visited. My wife, Marsha, would join me occasionally on the weekends and the three of us would sit around the table while the girls colored and horsed around on the furniture. When other family members visited on the weekends, this is where we took her as well.

Of course, Mom visited her every chance she could. This was the second benefit to me of having Mamaw in Bedford. It meant I got to see my mother a lot more than I normally did. I dearly love her and cherish all those extra times I got to see her during Mamaw's final years. We spent many days sitting around that table visiting with Mamaw and each other. We spent a lot of time reminiscing about the lakes and Mamaw's antics.

Mom recalled a story involving Amy. Amy was young, five or six at the time. Mom was sitting at the picnic table on the porch of Mamaw's trailer. Amy interrupted the conversation to tell Mom she was going swimming. Mom said okay and went back to her conversation. Whoever Mom had been talking to that day was stunned at what had happened. She asked Mom if Amy wasn't a little young to be swimming unsupervised. Mom grinned and told them to come with her. They stepped down from the porch and walked to the lake's edge where Amy was "swimming". There was Amy, standing a foot from shore where the water barely reached her ankles, using the pier like a table and playing with her dolls. Mom explained to them that Amy was terrified of water, and this was as far as she would dare to go. To her little mind, she was swimming because she was in the lake. They both had a good laugh over this.

Mom and I both had so many fond memories of Mamaw that we never ran out of stories. When Mamaw had visitors outside the immediate family, Mom usually came down so she could see them too. We ended up having many small reunions at Mamaw's new residence in Bedford.

She was loved by everyone and got lots of visitors that first year. All her other grandkids came at various times with their families. Her brother, my Uncle George, was driven to Bedford by Bryan to visit one time. Uncle George came down another time with her younger brother, my Uncle Phil. That was a great visit for us, seeing them together. Both of my uncles were in their late seventies or early eighties at that time. The two of them had recently completed a trip across the country in a pick-up truck with a camper shell over the bed. The two of them would take turns driving and at night, they would sleep on a mattress in the bed of the truck. I can't imagine taking on an adventure like that when I am in my seventies. Shoot, I can't imagine doing that at my age now! I could see those two laughing and joking the whole trip. Mamaw's nephew, Ronnie Craft, made several trips to visit with his Aunt Thelma. Ronnie was one of Aunt Isabelle's kids (Isabelle being Mamaw's sister). He was the only one of her nephews who saw Mamaw the most throughout her life. Ronnie was who she usually called if she had something mechanical that needed to be fixed. Ronnie also had a very small trailer at Pinkerton's Landing for a few years when I was young.

Uncle George was a carpenter with his own construction company, so she called him for problems with her home. She also called him one time about her teeth. She had broken her false teeth and for whatever reason, she had called Uncle George to come and take her to get them fixed. He showed up at her house and, with one look at her teeth, he told her he could fix them for her. I can just imagine that conversation:

"Thelma, you don't need to pay to fix your teeth. I'll fix them for you."

"How you going to fix my broken teeth, Bud?"

"Why, Thelma, all it needs is a little Super Glue and they'll be just like new."

"Super Glue? You can't fix teeth with Super Glue!"

"Sure you can! Super Glue fixes everything."

"Okay, if you say so, Bud."

I can see him taking the two broken pieces of her dentures in his big strong hands and slapping on a stream of Super Glue. He then would have held them firmly together while the glue set. After inspecting his work, he would have pulled out a piece of sandpaper and smoothed out the Super Glue on the surface. Once he was satisfied with his work, he would have handed them back to her, and said something like, "See, Thelma? You can't even tell they were broken now." This would have been followed by that deep, full-of-life laugh of his.

Her memory issues seemed unchanged those first few months. Or, at least, there was no noticeable major decline that I could see. It was hard to be sure because Mamaw was good at hiding the fact she couldn't remember names. She would greet people with terms of endearment, which was how she had always greeted people her entire life. Looking back, had I paid better attention, I might have realized she rarely used names in any of her conversations. Noticing this wouldn't have made any difference to her condition, though. Besides, I was more concerned with visiting with her and drawing her into conversations about anything and everything. The only real memory issue that was hard to miss was about her broken leg. She kept forgetting that it was broken and how she'd hurt it the entire six weeks it was in a cast. I answered the same questions countless times each visit:

"What's this big ole thing doing on my leg?" she'd ask.

"It's a cast, Mamaw. You broke your leg," I'd reply.

"Why did I do that?"

"It was an accident, Mamaw. You were at my house and fell."

"Oh, mercy me, I forgot about that. I'm sorry, sugar, I don't know why I keep forgetting that."

"That's okay, Mamaw. I wouldn't want to remember it either."

We'd get back to visiting for a while until she would try to move her leg again, which would lead to another round of "what's on my leg?"

"What's this big ole' thing on my leg?"

"It's a cast, Mamaw. You broke your leg…"

And I would have another variation of the conversation again. It didn't matter how many times she asked, I would always answer it the same way. I never lost my patience or got upset. It wasn't her fault she couldn't remember. Besides, she asked these questions so often that my responses were automatic. Her question about her leg was like a natural break in our conversation before we could move on to talking about something else. The only time she didn't ask as much was when the girls were with me. She loved watching them play and holding them on her lap. Jade particularly, who was still a baby.

Spring began approaching and I could bundle Mamaw up and take her outside now and then. Some days, I'd push her down the sidewalk and along the parking lot to the rear of the nursing home, and then back to the front entrance. The facility had a few rocking chairs out front. I liked to wheel her outside to them and sit beside her. We'd watch the birds and squirrels across the streets. I did most of the talking. At first, I had the misguided belief that I could make her remember things. I thought if I talked about the different memories I had from growing up with her I could make her remember. If I could get her to remember, then maybe it would slow down the dementia.

I knew this was only wishful thinking on my part, and not sensible. I think everyone who must deal with a loved one stricken with dementia goes through this phase. I imagine the experts would say it's a natural part of a denial phase we all go through when we first deal with this horrible affliction. This may be a typical reaction, but it is not good for your loved one. Pressuring them to remember events can agitate them and, even worse, scare them. Nothing good can come from making them realize they are forgetting things. The best way to deal with this is to make sure they are comfortable and visit with them regularly.

The initial stages of dementia involve short-term memory loss, and people start forgetting simple things. In Mamaw's case, it was getting disoriented at Lake Erie. Then it was the lighting of cigarettes and finding her way home. As dementia's grip tightens on them, they start losing memories of the past and forgetting names of friends and acquaintances. It ultimately steals their memories of immediate family members, their children, and grandchildren. As horrible and painful as this is to witness, they still retain a large part of their personality. My sister had some wonderful visits with Mamaw, even though she had no idea she was her granddaughter. They laughed and talked about everything. It was the same with all my conversations with her. She was still Mamaw. Everything she said and did was the same as it always had been with her. She could make me laugh, even if she had no clue who I was because she was still Mamaw.

It didn't matter that my stories had no effect on her regaining her memory. And, it certainly didn't matter if she remembered anything from whatever story I was telling her. My stories were good for both of us. I could stroll down memory lane, where I had a lifetime of good memories of Mamaw, Mom, and my brothers and sisters to talk about. It was good for her because I know she enjoyed listening to me as I made those journeys through time. She'd laugh at the funny parts, saying, "Oh my!" at the right spots. Now and then, she would reward me with a remark that made it clear I had triggered some memory she still had. She would say something like, "Oh, that Scotty was something," or "How is my Sherry Kay?" For a moment, I knew she had found that small island of memories and remembered something or someone.

I never tried to force the issue of getting her to remember anything specific. I would ask her if she remembered some event, but no matter what her answer was, I would still launch into a story about it. I didn't want to make her feel bad if she didn't remember something. I think the real reason was more selfish. I didn't want to know when she had forgotten something because it reminded me of her dementia and I avoided those thoughts as much as I could. For many of my visits that first year, I became a storyteller to an audience of one. The two of us would escape for an hour or so each day to whatever places my memories took us. Precious memories to me, and good stories to her.

I might tell her something like, "I was thinking about that family vacation we all took to Lake Erie the other day. Do you remember that vacation, Mamaw?" She'd say no or that she wasn't sure. I'd start talking about it anyway, telling her the story about my favorite family vacation.

Mom was there. All Mamaw's grandkids were came with their families: me and Marsha, Scott and Shannon, Laura and her husband, James and Lisa, Amy and Aaron, and all her great-grandkids. Aunt Frances and Rex were on that vacation too. Oh, how we laughed sitting on the porch of one of the cabins playing the card game Spoons, Sequence, or Uno for hours and hours. Age never mattered in our family. Anyone who wanted to play could join in. Mamaw always played. I loved those family gatherings. We always had an enjoyable time when we got the family together.

That was the vacation when we played that silly ball game Mom had brought. It had this goofy pink and yellow cap with rows of Velcro strips running from the front to back. The cap fit on your head like the hood part of a sweatshirt. There were about ten balls that were made of a rough cloth that stuck to Velcro, and they were thrown at the person wearing the hood. Mom split everyone up into groups of two and we took turns seeing who could get the most balls stuck on the other person's hooded head. It was the silliest game, and we all laughed as we watched each other running around like fools trying to make the balls stick to the cap. I remember seeing how much Mamaw was enjoying the whole spectacle. Mom did too and asked her if she wanted to play. We were all shocked when Mamaw said she did.

I quickly volunteered to be her partner. I tied that silly hat on her head, then backed up a short distance to lob the balls at her. I tried hard to toss them as close to her head as possible so she wouldn't have to move much. It didn't matter, though, because she had some competitive juices kick in and acted like she wanted to win the game. She ran back and forth, bobbing and weaving her head, trying hard to catch those balls. She was moving like a teenager instead of a woman in her eighties. The entire family was laughing so hard seeing Mamaw running around like she was still a kid. She was giving it her all to catch those silly balls. Whenever she did catch one, we all cheered and clapped in excitement.

When I had thrown the last ball, I asked her if she was all right. She said she was. I then picked up all the balls that had missed and stuck them all over her head and we posed together for a picture.

60

I had an eight-by-ten picture made of this, and have it prominently displayed in my house.

Yep, that vacation was one of my favorites.

After I told her the story, I looked at her and could tell she had enjoyed it by the smile on her face. I had no idea whether she remembered it or not, but it didn't matter. The story had done its job and taken us both to a happy place. I knew that it was extremely important for me not to push her to remember the different stories I'd tell her. The only thing that would have accomplished was it might make her feel bad for not remembering or, God forbid, it might remind her there was something wrong with her. No, these stories were more for my benefit as I traveled down memory lane. To her, they were simply happy stories being told to her.

Spring's approach brought about a few more good things. Mamaw's cast got to come off and she began her physical therapy. During the next few months, I tried to be there every day for her therapy to encourage her.

With the warmer weather of spring, I could also wheel her out in the courtyard when I had the girls with me. I always brought a bag of carrots so the girls could feed the rabbits. I would put Mamaw in charge of them, so the girls had to go to her when they needed another carrot. She enjoyed giving carrots to the girls and watching them running around chasing the rabbits or trying to lure them close to catch one. I never worried about them catching the rabbits because they were fast. Boy, was I wrong! Mamaw and I were discussing something and weren't paying very close attention to the girls. Sage waddled up to the patio carrying a rabbit that was half her size and too heavy for her to hold. She had a strained look on her face when she said, "Look, Papaw, I caught a rabbit." I never knew how she managed to catch it, but it was a one-time incident because she was never able to catch another.

Jade was starting to walk by this time, but she wasn't very stable on her feet yet. I would hold her hand and walk her out to a safe place in the grass so she could feed the rabbits. I'd break off a piece of carrot and hand it to her to throw. She'd haul that little arm back and throw that carrot as hard as she could, sending it sailing through the air to land a few feet in front of her. She'd clap her little hands and then wobble back to me for another piece. When we needed another carrot, she would grab my hand and lead me to

Mamaw for another one. Back and forth we all went until Mamaw ran out of carrots. She always sounded truly sad when she'd have to tell those little girls, "All gone."

Sometimes, I would carry the bag to the edge of the courtyard and stand in one place while breaking off pieces for the girls. We would toss all the carrots to the center of the courtyard, then return to Mamaw. Together, we would all wait to see how many rabbits were lured out of their underground hiding spots for the carrot buffet we had made. This was a game we played, to see what the highest number of rabbits was that could be seen out in the courtyard at one time. For a while, Mamaw would help the girls by searching and pointing at rabbits when she saw them. Another precious memory I'll always cherish.

Mamaw could get around with a walker about the time the weather got nice enough, and we would spend most of my visits outside. Eventually, her leg got strong enough she could walk the hallways on her own with her walker, which opened the whole nursing home to her. This helped her recovery a lot, and it was no time before she could walk without the walker. For a while, she had to walk along the wall and hold the handrail, but before long, she was walking those hallways down the middle, lap after lap. She spent most of her days walking around those hallways, greeting everyone she passed, every time she passed them. In the afternoons, she would eat lunch, go for a few more laps, and then lie down and take a nap for an hour or so as part of her daily routine.

Easter of that year, we decided to have a huge celebration at my house for Mamaw's benefit, while she could still enjoy a family gathering. It was also done for everyone else's benefit because we knew her condition was only going to get worse. I had a large house outside Bedford city limits with enough space to accommodate the party. I brought in extra tables and set them up on my covered front porch for dining. Uncle George came with Bryan and Marta. Marta's husband, Rusty, and Bryan's wife Rosie attended as well. And, of course, the entire extended Kern clan made sure to come to this gathering.

Mamaw loved living at the nursing home and was happy. The time arrived when her recovery was complete and Mom needed to start considering moving her out of the nursing home. She brought the subject up with me and we discussed the choices she had. Taking her back to Laura's house wasn't an option anymore because it would only be a short-term solution. Moving her to a nursing home closer to Mom was the best scenario for Mom because she could spend more time with Mamaw if she were closer. I wanted Mamaw kept where she was, and told Mom this. I reminded her that Mamaw had been up north, closer to everyone else in the family except me, for my entire adult life. Each of them got to visit and spend time with her a lot more often than I could after I left home for the Army and then moved to Bedford (except for Scott, who had moved to Atlanta, Georgia). When Mamaw's dementia first affected her life, they got to take care of her because they lived closer to her. I told Mom it was my turn with Mamaw, and she agreed to leave her in Bedford.

Selfish reasons aside, it was the choice that made the most sense. I had the flexibility with work. The nursing home was located on my route to and from work. But the most important reason was that Mamaw enjoyed being there. The staff loved her, and she was gaining weight. Mom began the process of making her home at the facility permanent. This involved selling her few assets, as is required by Medicare for long-term care. The proceeds had to go into an account that would pay for her stay, and Medicare would take care of the bills once the account was emptied.

That first year in the nursing home, Mamaw was very happy. She had her routines. She continued to participate in Bingo and other activities the facility put on. She loved it when people came and sang for the residents, especially when they sang the old gospel songs and the old country and western songs. She always got to see one face she remembered every day because of my visits, and she got a steady stream of family members stopping in.

My cousin Penny came to see Mamaw, along with her family. Mamaw's nephew, Ronnie, was the most frequent out-of-town visitor. He'd show up out of the blue. I would go to visit her and there was Ronnie. Considering how far Bedford was from most of the family, she was blessed to have so many people make the drive to see her. Of course, she was a special lady to many people.

Chapter 7
The Demon Tightens His Grip

Mom has always come to my house for Thanksgiving every year and celebrated with my family. That first year Mamaw was in the nursing home, I brought her to the house for the entire day. Laura and her family came to town and joined us, along with Marsha's mother, Dottie. Dottie had one of her friends come that year, and Mamaw seemed to enjoy visiting with her. They talked like they had known each other their whole lives. Of course, Mamaw thought they had. And it wasn't only on holidays that I brought her to the house. If Mom could make it into town for the weekend, we always brought Mamaw out for a day during these times as well.

Mamaw's life was now regimented, which was a good thing. It's important that people with memory issues have routines to make sure their daily lives are familiar to them, lessening the risk of confusing them. I tried not to disrupt her routines. If she were asleep when I arrived, I would leave and return later. If she were out for a walk, I would join her, greeting the people with her as we passed them, each time we passed them.

We broke her daily routine once that first summer. We knew how she felt about being near water, and Mom thought it would be nice to bring her out to her house on Cordry Lake for a family gathering and cookout. I picked Mamaw up in my van and took her with my family. The drive was only about an hour, and we made it most of the way when Mamaw started getting agitated. Marsha talked with her and calmed her down for the remainder of the drive.

Mamaw did all right for most of the time at Mom's house, visiting with everyone and enjoying the lake view. As it got later, she started getting nervous and remarking that she needed to get home. Mom thought we should do what she wanted. I loaded Mamaw into the van and headed back to Bedford. Mamaw was a nervous wreck the whole way home. I didn't think I was going to be able to get her back in time, and had no idea what to do as a backup plan. It took my entire family working together to get her back. Marsha and the kids talked with her and tried to keep her distracted and calm. They had to do this the entire drive back to the nursing home. We never tried to take Mamaw on a road trip again after that.

I didn't even try to bring her over to my house after this, for fear of scaring or upsetting her.

Things went well for a while after this. I kept visiting and telling her stories from my time growing up with her. I continued to bring the girls whenever I could and loaded up the whole family regularly to visit with her as well. Since I was around her every day and she was used to my voice, she always recognized me, right up to the very end. She knew I was her grandson for quite some time and always recognized me by my voice. I never observed any serious decline in her memory for some time because of this.

Our daughter, Amber, drove to Bedford one Saturday right after her first child, Blake, was born. Mamaw could still hold Blake, and she did for quite a long time. It was so adorable the way she cradled him in her frail arms, rubbing his little cheeks and talking to him. Dottie was with us that day. Marsha and Sage and Jade were present as well. Naturally, we got some rabbit time in, which made everyone happy. That was a good day for Mamaw.

It was when other family members visited that it became obvious the dementia was gradually getting worse. Laura would come up for a day and spend hours visiting with her. Mamaw would introduce her to people as her good friend, seeing her as some person from her past, rather than the granddaughter she lovingly called Laurie. Uncle George came back, and she had no idea who he was at first, but soon she recognized him. I remember James and Lisa coming down to see her with their sons Reed and Tate, and I don't think she recognized any of them. This was tough for me to see when she didn't recognize any of her other grandkids. But the worst was when she started forgetting my Mom. This broke my heart.

The first time I witnessed it, Mom had come to visit and she greeted Mamaw with her usual happiness, saying, "Hi, Mom!" Mamaw looked towards her with a confused expression. Without missing a beat, Mom said, "Come on, Mom, you remember me, Sherry Kay." I could see the change come over Mamaw's face as she found that thread of memory and grabbed hold of it, and then she said, "Of course, I remember you, pumpkin." And I knew she did. But it wasn't much longer before she couldn't remember, and it tore me up.

I knew how much she loved and adored my mother, and when she lost that memory of her was when the reality of her dementia slammed home with me. I had to look away as I fought back tears for what I knew my mom had to be feeling right then. But my mom is one of the strongest people I know, and she had known this day would come. She hid whatever she was feeling and reacted like Mamaw knew her and kissed her on the cheek, then struck up a conversation like everything was fine. She is one special lady, my mom, and I was blessed to have her. Of course, she'd had one special mom as well.

Mom bought Mamaw a recliner so she would have something comfortable to sit in during the day. At first, the nursing home refused to put her in it because they were afraid she might fall out of it. Mom spoke to someone and convinced them that this was hogwash, and got them to start putting her in it every morning. I would have loved to be a fly on the wall during that conversation. I think Mamaw enjoyed spending most of her time each day sitting in her recliner. It wasn't unusual for me to stop by and find her frail little body sound asleep in that huge chair. I found it reassuring to see that her recliner had the same effect on her as mine did on me.

I continued with my routine of coming to see her every day, and Mamaw stuck to hers. One day while she was making her usual rounds through the hallways, performing her daily resident greeting duties, she forgot where her room was. People with dementia don't ask for help when they're scared. Disorientation quickly leads to fear with them. The natural thing for Mamaw to do would have been to keep looking for her room. That's exactly what she did too. She walked those hallways, lap after lap, around and around those same corridors, over and over until she was completely exhausted. Tired, lost, scared, and alone. She wandered into a hallway that had just been mopped and slipped on the wet floor, breaking her arm. It hurts to think of how long she must have walked those halls. Walking all alone without any of the staff realizing she need help finding her room. Her fear would certainly have put a look of distress on her face. Exhaustion would have slowed her down and made her noticeably sluggish as she walked. I am sure the overwhelming fatigue she encountered would have caused her to shuffle and slide her feet. Yet, no one noticed.

I can only pray she didn't lay there, helpless and in severe pain, for too long. Oh, how I pray someone on the staff heard her painful cries for help right away. It breaks my heart to think of her lying on the floor, all alone and confused. Somebody did find her, and the nursing home had her taken by ambulance to the hospital for X-rays.

This break was serious and required surgery as well. Sure enough, the surgery couldn't be done until the next day. I wasn't about to leave her alone for the night. I had a pretty good idea of what to expect this time around. I convinced them to let her keep her panties on, so at least I wouldn't be having *that* conversation again. I still had to deal with the lights coming on all night and upsetting her, but it didn't take much effort to calm her down. They had her sedated much more this time.

Morning arrived, and they prepped her for surgery. They had given her something to help her relax through her IV while she was still in her hospital room. She was snoring as they wheeled her bed towards the operating room. I walked with them through the hallway, remaining by her side, more for my own comfort than for any other reason. We had to stop in the hallway and wait a few minutes before they were ready to take her in for surgery.

While she lay on the gurney, knocked out from the sedative, I watched as she raised one hand to her face. She then placed her mouth between the pointer and middle finger and took a deep imaginary puff. She then lowered her hand while blowing out an imaginary plume of smoke. I guess it doesn't matter how long it's been since a person last smoked, in some far recess of the brain, it remembers the addiction. She had smoked her whole life, and the anesthesia somehow took her back to a time when she smoked. So, there she was, lying on the hospital gurney, out like a light and smoking an imaginary cigarette. I couldn't help but smile as I stood beside her while she took one puff after another. She looked so peaceful without any signs of stress or worry on her face. I knew that wherever her dreams had taken her, it must have been a happy memory for her. The surgery was successful and she went to recovery with another cast to deal with, this time on her arm.

Mamaw was soon transported back to the nursing home, where I was waiting for her once again. She surprised me and was taking this well, which was a relief. Her arm was placed in a sling, to help her to lug that heavy cast around on her arm. She may have been gaining weight, but she was still very frail. She didn't let the weight of the cast keep her from her hallway walks, however, and was back at it in no time. Mom was walking with her one day, right after she'd broken her arm, and noticed Mamaw seemed to be having a difficult time breathing. She knew right away there was something wrong. The weight of the cast wasn't enough to cause the degree of difficulty she was having. She contacted Mamaw's doctor right away and told him of this change. When he arrived, and listened to her lungs, he called an ambulance to come and take her to the emergency room without delay.

He had tests run and found a huge mass on her lungs. She had cancer. There was no sign of the mass on the X-rays that had been taken a few years earlier, and based on the size of the mass, it was growing fast. The doctor said surgery was an option but he couldn't make any guarantees it would rid her of the cancer. Mamaw was 89 years old, so Mom didn't mince words with him. She asked him straight up, "Based on her age, how long would she likely have without the surgery, and how much time would the surgery give her?"

The doctor said, "Without surgery, she likely only has about six months to live. With surgery, she might have a year."

This made the decision a little easier for Mom. I shouldn't say easier because there is nothing easy about having to decide on something this serious. But Mom didn't want to put her through the surgery and the recovery. It was more important to her, and to us, that Mamaw be kept comfortable her remaining time. Dementia was already taking her from us. Why make her fight another demon? Mamaw was returned to the nursing home none the wiser, and we went about things like we had before this heavy news.

Mamaw had the same issues with this cast as she'd had with her broken leg, and was continually forgetting what had happened to her arm.

"Why's this thing on my arm?"

"You broke your arm, Mamaw."

"I did? Why did I do that?"

"It was an accident, Mamaw. You were out for a walk and slipped and fell. You broke your arm. Does it hurt?"

"No, not really. Did they have to put this heavy thing on it?"

"Yes, they did, Mamaw. They don't want you to hurt it again while the bone heals."

69

"Okay, sweetie. It is heavy, though. Look, I can't lift my arm up."

"I know, Mamaw. Don't do that. You need to leave it down until it heals."

"Okay, honey, if you say so."

I would have similar conversations with her multiple times a day, every day of the week, until the cast was removed.

I tried to increase my visits as much as I could so I could take her outside or to a window somewhere, to give her something more pleasant to look at. Marsha would bring our kids, Bobby and Robby, and our granddaughters, Sage and Jade, to see her more often after she got home from work. It was important to me that all the kids spend as much time with Mamaw as they could. Mamaw loved visitors, and when the girls came to see her she always perked up. She enjoyed watching everything they did, smiling the whole time they were there. As soon as they found out where they were going, the first thing they asked was if we could take Mamaw outside to see the rabbits.

I'm certain she no longer recognized the boys as her great grandkids or the girls as her great-great-grandkids, but that didn't matter. These visits served a different purpose for each of us, and whether she recognized anybody was of no significance. Our kids were adults by then and were fortunate to have already experienced plenty of great memories with Mamaw while they were growing up. They were good about sitting and visiting with her when they were with me. Bobby and Robby would play cards with her during many of their earlier visits when she could do so. She was still able to communicate with them, even when she could no longer play cards, which made it easier for them. She would respond and even ask them questions. It didn't bother either of them that her eyes were always drawn to whatever Sage and Jade were doing.

After what seemed life forever, Mamaw got the cast off, and that's when I started noticing more of a change in her from the dementia. Mom and everyone else could see the decline in her mental capacities a lot sooner because they weren't with her every day. It was different for me. We had our own routines we went through. We roamed around the halls and the parking lot. We sat and visited in the visitor's area and on the front porch. We fed the rabbits with the girls. And I continued talking to Mamaw like I always had, like nothing was wrong with her. I kept telling her stories, hoping to bring her with me on my journeys down memory lane. Each day I saw her, she seemed the same as she had the previous day.

Being with her so often and for so long, I could anticipate her needs without realizing I was doing so. I waited on her, and pampered her, in my efforts to make sure she was comfortable. I think this continual contact and interaction between us buffered me from many of the signs that the dementia was getting worse. I saw her every day, and wouldn't have noticed slight changes anyway. I was slowly doing more and more for her without realizing it. I was too busy taking care of her to notice this. It kept me from worrying unnecessarily about her deteriorating health. It's possible that I didn't notice any changes in her condition because I didn't want to see it. This would have forced me to confront the reality of the situation. Whatever the reason, I was very happy being with her all those times.

My visits with her were precious, and I always looked forward to entering her room and seeing her lying in her bed. It always brought a joyous smile to my face when I entered the nursing home and spotted her sitting outside her door, or when I'd find her after roaming the hallways, if she was out on one of her walks. Every time I laid my eyes on her, my heart lifted and a smile would find its way to my face, washing away all the stress of the day. All my life, Mamaw had this effect on me. It was like all those times Marta took me skiing at Dewart Lake. The high point of skiing was each time she took the boat along the shore where our trailer was. I'd start scanning the shoreline to find our trailer and Mamaw sitting at her spot on the porch. Once I found her, I would wave like a madman to get her attention until she waved back at me. Spotting her in the nursing home gave me the same feeling of happiness as when she would notice me skiing and stand up to return my wave. This was exactly why I loved showing up unannounced at her home and work. She never lost this effect on me.

All my life, she always acted the same. There was nothing fake about her, or about my mother, for that matter. They were both the most genuine people I knew. All my memories of Mamaw were precious. They were fun. They were happy. To me, she encompassed everything that was good in life. Whenever she saw me, her reaction was sincere. She was truly happy to see me. So, when I laid my eyes on her, I always felt this. I saw her as she had always been to me. My mamaw. And it never failed to make me happy.

I honestly don't think I ever thought about her dying, even though I knew the dementia would, in time, take her from me.

Eventually, she became noticeably different even to me. It was shortly after she had recovered from her broken arm that I could no longer deny seeing her decline. She started becoming a little less responsive when interacting with me. She started sleeping more and appearing lethargic when I visited. She got to where she couldn't get out of bed by herself, and the nurses had to get her up and into her recliner. Worst of all, she wasn't eating as much as normal and started to lose weight she didn't have to lose. She was still able to feed herself for a while. The problem was that she wasn't eating as much at each meal. The nurses were required to document what the residents consumed at each meal, so when Mamaw started eating less, one of them would sit down and coax her to eat more. They started including a carton of some sort of vitamin supplement shake as part of her meals, which she liked. When Mom learned about this change, she and I made sure she always had a supply of Ensure in her room like we did with her snacks. This helped stop the weight loss and she started gaining a little back.

Her memory loss got so bad that the nursing staff was concerned about her roaming off. They decided to remove her bed and had her sleeping on a mattress on the floor. Then they connected her to an alarm, so they would get alerted if she ever got up. The alarm was a little cord that wrapped around her waist and plugged into an alarm. If she got up, the cord would disconnect from the plug, setting off an alarm at the nurse's station. They had a problem with her frequently setting the alarm off and contacted Mom about it. They wanted permission to strap her into bed at night, to keep her from getting up. Mom told them, "Absolutely not," and made a trip to the nursing home to visit Mamaw and address the alarm issue. Right away, she realized the problem. The nursing home had removed Mamaw's bed and moved the mattress up against the wall. The side that Mamaw was used to sleeping on was now facing the wall, and this confused her. The confusion made her disoriented, and scared her a bit, causing her to get up. This was a perfectly normal reaction for her if she didn't know where she was. Mom had them return the bed to her room and place it back in its original position.

Problem solved. Mamaw no longer tried getting out of bed in the middle of the night and set off the alarm.

This is a prime example of how professional caregivers need to consider the residents and patients first when making changes that affect them. Somewhere along the line, somebody should have seen and remembered which side Mamaw slept on at night. Most people have a favorite position or side they sleep on. Habits that have been ingrained in a person's behavior their whole life aren't going to change because a person has dementia. The incident of Mamaw smoking an imaginary cigarette when she was sedated proves that long-term behaviors are permanently imprinted in our brains and don't simply go away. The nurses hadn't taken the time to consider this decision all the way through from Mamaw's perspective. At no time did one of them even consider which way she faced when she slept. Routines are important to patients with memory issues. Every decision made by professional caregivers and by family members should begin with the question "How is this going to affect the patient?" It's irresponsible to decide from the point of "What is the most convenient thing for me?"

Chapter 8
My First Loss to Dementia

My father-in-law, David Lyons, was my first experience of losing someone close to me to dementia. Losing him was hard for us, especially Marsha and her mother Dottie. Seeing this horrible disease grab hold of David and slowly take him away from us was heartbreaking. Alzheimer's causes dementia, so what he went through was very much like what Mamaw experienced. I can recall his regression as that disease progressed. Seeing the first symptoms of him losing his short-term memory and then started getting lost and disoriented. Then he got to where he couldn't recognize anyone. Over time came the slow loss of bodily control.

David was born and raised in Bedford, Indiana. His father was a fire and brimstone Nazarene preacher who traveled the area doing tent revivals. His mother was a full-blooded Cherokee Indian. As a teenager, he used to sell ice cream from a bicycle around town. The bike had two wheels in front to support the large wooden box that held the ice cream. The rest of the bike was behind the ice cream box. The bicycle frame and seat, a single tire, and the handlebars were mounted on the wooden box. Basically, it was like riding a tricycle backward while pushing a trailer. Bedford had another teenager in town who also sold ice cream from a bike. According to David, it was a fierce competition between them as each tried to beat the other to the various hotspots for selling their treats. The other young man's name was Claude Akins.

Claude would go on to become a television and movie star. His film career included roles in some classic movies with some of the biggest names in Hollywood. His films included; *From Here to Eternity* with Burt Lancaster, Frank Sinatra, Montgomery Cliff, and Deborah Kerr; *The Caine Mutiny* with Humphrey Bogart, Fred MacMurray, Lee Marvin; and *Rio Bravo* with John Wayne and Dean Martin. He appeared in dozens of television shows, including many old westerns like *The Rifleman, Rawhide, Gunsmoke*, and *Bonanza*. He was most well-known for his role as the sheriff in *BJ and the Bear*, a show about the adventures of a truck driver and his traveling companion, a chimpanzee named Bear.

Dottie was born in Chicago, Illinois. Her father was Anthony Russo, an Italian man with ties to the mob in Chicago. He owned a few bars that dated back to the days of prohibition. Her mother, Anna Ruth Russo, was also Italian and she had five sisters.

Work was hard to find in Bedford when David was a young man. He headed for Chicago with his best friend Irvin Armstrong to take a job trimming trees. He was at a county carnival one night when Dottie spotted him. David liked to tell people how she was smitten with him and kept throwing popcorn at him to get his attention. Dottie never denied it. She would always grin and say he looked like Burt Lancaster in the movie *From Here to Eternity* when he was at the carnival. It's funny how of all the movies and movie stars she would see a resemblance to a star in a movie his ice cream nemesis was in. They married and were inseparable from then on.

They weren't in Chicago long before moving back to Bedford so David could take a job at General Motors. They would have two daughters, Valerie and Marsha. After some time, David would retire from General Motors. A couple of years later we would get the terrible news that David had Alzheimer's and dementia. The disease progressed much fast with David than any of us were prepared for.

Dottie chose to keep him at home, and we visited them multiple times each week. David was a tall, husky man, and I would help her pull him up to a standing position from his recliner. I would watch her guide him to the bedroom, where Marsha would help undress him and get him into his pajamas. Then the two of them would coax him to lie down in their bed. I could only imagine how difficult it was for this little Italian woman, who somehow managed to get him to stand up from his recliner by herself, over and over, day after day. Of course, we would do anything for those we loved, no matter how painful to our own bodies and minds, and I know she never regretted her decision to care for him herself.

Dottie kept David home for nearly the entire time while this demonic disease stole the man she had loved her whole life away from her. We helped as often as we could, but she shouldered the brunt of the responsibilities by herself. I have such admiration for the way she took care of him, and especially for how long she managed to do it. Her reward was that she got to be with the love of her life every moment, right up to near the end. It didn't matter at all to her that he didn't know who she was those last few years. It never bothered her that he shuffled like a zombie when she guided him around the house, or that she had to feed him every meal. It didn't matter at all to her that he had to wear a diaper when he could no longer control his bodily functions. She had to clean him up and change him throughout the day, never once complaining. I have no doubt it was worth every sacrifice and every painstaking task because she got to be near him. She could hold his hand, kiss his cheek, and hug him whenever she wanted. She got to lie next to this man every night and wake up with him beside her every morning. She got to spend every minute of every day with the man whom she had fallen in love with, made a life and family with, and grown old with. I am confident that she felt the sacrifices she made for him were more than worth what she got in return. How could I not admire someone who would do this?

David stayed with her nearly to the end. After some time, he got to where he no longer reacted to her directions. It became impossible for her to get him to eat. Dottie was forced to reconsider her decision to care for him at home when she couldn't get him to move at all. He was too heavy for her to lift when he became nonresponsive. God love her, she tried for as long as she could, before tearfully making the decision to have him placed in a nursing home. This nearly broke her heart. She still spent every waking moment by his side. She only left for errands if Marsha or I came to her house to be with him in her absence. David wasn't in the nursing home very long before succumbing to this awful disease and joining God in heaven. He died quietly in his sleep on December 19, 1998. We were blessed and got to be with him early in the evening before he died. For the first time in a long time, he was awake and responsive while we were with him. Marsha got him to eat his supper that evening, a bowl of chili.

Having witnessed this with David, I knew exactly what to expect with Mamaw's diagnosis. I just never thought about it. I don't think this was intentional. Of course, I didn't want her to die. I didn't block this from my mind or make a conscious effort to avoid thinking about it. No, I was guided by love to take care of my Mamaw, like Dottie had been with David. She was always a huge part of my life. When she was admitted to the nursing home it only seemed right that I visit her every day. I didn't want her to ever feel alone and wanted to make sure she could see a familiar face. I talked to her and treated her with love like I always had, not because I knew I would lose her.

Chapter 9
Happy 90ᵗʰ Birthday, Mamaw

Once Mamaw's condition had declined to where she needed help getting up and down, and with everything else, the nursing home moved her to their full-care wing. This wing was down at the end of her current hallway, but instead of turning right to go to the main cafeteria, her room was in the hallway to the left. The full-care wing had a smaller dining room for its residents. This worked for a bit, but dementia is an evil demon and once those talons have a person firmly in their grip, it takes more and more from a person. Stripping them of their memories isn't enough. It deprives them of their ability to function, stealing their humanity from them. It wasn't long before Mamaw stopped feeding herself.

I frequently stopped by at meal times, when she was still eating in the larger dining room and would visit with her and the other folks at her table while she ate. The first time I came to visit her in the new dining room, I wasn't happy at all with what I saw. The nurses that were feeding other residents weren't paying attention to them, barely even speaking. They sat next to them feeding them like babies, except I couldn't hear any encouragement being spoken to get them to eat. It seemed to me that it was more of a chore to them – a task that needed completion, and nothing more. When it came time for Mamaw to eat, they brought her tray to the table and I politely told them I would feed her.

I sat with her, feeding her one bite at a time, talking to her with each bite.

"Okay, Mamaw, let's try a bite of this chocolate pudding. You like chocolate pudding, and this actually looks pretty good."

And she'd open her mouth and take a bite. And another, and then another, until it was all gone.

I would continue to ramble on and on while I fed her, to keep her distracted.

"See? I knew you'd like that. Now, let's try this meat. I think it's meatloaf, but I'm not sure. Do you think this looks like meatloaf? I don't know, maybe it's Salisbury steak. What do you think? It smells good. Here, try it."

She would open her mouth and I would feed her, one bite at a time until that was gone. I didn't get her to eat everything, but I have a feeling she ate more of that meal than she had eaten in quite some time. From this point on, I tried to be with her for every meal she had, every single day. I did not want my Mamaw to be fed like a baby, and I was not going to allow someone to force food into her mouth like it was a chore. Spending time with her every day had made her recognize me as a friendly face. I also believe, from talking to her as much as I did, that she recognized my voice. This made her feel safe listening to me and made it easier for me to get her to eat. Then again, maybe she was sick of my nonstop chatter and only ate to get me to shut up. Seriously, though, she was eating and that made me feel better.

I started scheduling and planning my days around Mamaw's meals. I was an early riser, which helped a lot. I always have been since my time in the Army. I would go straight to the nursing home and feed her breakfast before heading in to open my business at 8 AM. I took a lunch break when it was time for her lunch, and when the store closed at 5 PM, I drove straight to the nursing home to feed her supper. Everybody on staff knew I did this, and I'm sure they appreciated having one less mouth to feed. They always left her tray in the warmer for me to take out when I got there. They had name labels on each tray, so all I had to do was search through them for Mamaw's. When she finished, I had to show her tray to a nurse so they could document what she had eaten before I could place it on the return tray rack.

It went on like this for a few months. I continued talking to Mamaw about whatever came to mind while I fed her whatever I could get her to eat. If I couldn't make it for a meal, I always let the nurses know ahead of time so they wouldn't wait and then feed her last, but I rarely missed one. I was too worried about the way the nurses fed her, and that she wouldn't eat if I wasn't there. My schedule was so flexible that I didn't have any problems making time for her.

With Mamaw's condition worsening so much, Mom decided it would be a good idea to have a birthday party for Mamaw for her ninetieth birthday. She wanted everybody to be able to get together for Mamaw, most likely for the last time. I think she also did it for Mamaw, hoping she could enjoy the family gathering before dementia dug its deadly claws into her any deeper. It was a great idea and turned out to be a wonderful day for everyone.

The nursing home let us use their parking lot in the back for the party. I used a delivery truck I had and picked up some banquet tables and chairs from the Stonehenge Lodge, a hotel in Bedford I had recently left after managing it for thirteen years. Mom bought a lot of the food, but everyone brought more items, turning it into quite the feast. The time came to get Mamaw and bring her out, so I went and got her. The nursing home had started putting her in a reclining chair on wheels every morning when she got up. I only had to push her outside for the party. Mom had picked out a spot in the shade under a tree for her where she would be comfortable sitting for the whole party. All the kids, grandkids, and great-grandkids showed up. This was no surprise to me. We thought so much of Mamaw that nothing could have kept any of us from being present. Uncle George, Uncle Phil, and my cousin Diana even managed to come. Mamaw slept most of the time she was outside, but when she was awake there was always someone sitting by her side talking to her.

Every single person took the time to sit by her and talk to her that day. Mom invited all the nurses on her wing to come out and grab some food and cake. I think every one of them found the time to come outside and wish Mamaw a happy birthday. I'm certain she didn't recognize anybody that day. The dementia demon had stolen all her memories by then. It still must have been an enjoyable day for her, with all the attention showered on her when she was awake and the festive atmosphere around her the whole time. At least I'd like to believe she could sense all the happy vibes. I do know it was a great day for everyone else. It was like one of our family reunions from the past. Everyone got to give Mamaw hugs and kisses as many times as they wanted. She may not have recognized anyone, but every person there could leave that day with the comforting knowledge that they got to see her one final time. They got to tell her goodbye. After a while, the party ended and the last of the family left, and Mamaw was pushed back to her room.

Chapter 10
An Angel Gets Her Wings

The demon was tightening its grip on Mamaw, and she continued to lose more and more of herself to the beast of dementia. Mom had a mission trip to Jamaica coming up that she had been planning for some time. She was going to be working with some friends she'd met through her church to help build a church and school there. She came to visit Mamaw before leaving. After spending most of the day with her, she leaned over and kissed Mamaw on the cheek and hugged her. While she was hugging her, she leaned in close to Mamaw's ear and said, "Mom, I'm going to Jamaica and won't be able to visit you for a while." Something about this moment between mother and daughter resonated with Mamaw, pushing the demon back long enough for a moment of clarity. She looked into Mom's eyes with recognition. Mamaw then raised one hand up and began patting her cheek and said, "Okay, you be careful, sweetie."

This was the last time Mom would see her mother.

It became harder and harder for me to get Mamaw to eat solid foods. She would still eat ice cream for me, and when I put the straw from her shake in her mouth she would drink it. I had them start putting two shakes and two ice creams on her meal trays so she would get something in her system. I still tried to get her to eat some of the food on her tray. But, by this time, she couldn't chew. Hospice was called in, as required by the nursing homes, to help families prepare for the unavoidable loss of their loved one at this stage.

The woman assigned to Mamaw seemed aloof and cold to me. She talked to me a few times but I didn't listen. I wasn't ready to talk about Mamaw dying and took offense to this woman insisting we talk about it. I told her I didn't need her help preparing for this. I am sure I wasn't polite to her, and she was probably glad she wasn't going to have to deal with me. I regret the way I treated her, as she was simply doing her job. In my state of mind at the time, however, I didn't want anybody "helping" me get ready to lose Mamaw. I had been with her so much I didn't think I needed some stranger coming in and telling me what she did and didn't need. And I certainly didn't want to talk to her about Mamaw dying. I didn't want to talk to anybody about this. I continued with my routines, trying not to think about losing her.

It wasn't long before she wouldn't eat the ice cream, and I knew the shakes would be next. The brain controls everything, and eventually, the disease finds its way to the part of the brain that controls eating and drinking. I think I could get her to drink the shakes even after her brain had forgotten how to eat because drinking was some form of reflex memory. As soon as her mouth felt the tip of the straw on her lips, she instinctively put it in her mouth and began drinking, but what little nutrition she got from those shakes wasn't enough to sustain her body. I was begging her at every meal to drink for me. I'd say, "Come on, Mamaw, please take another drink for me," or, "Please, Mamaw, please. Just a little more. That's all. Please, Mamaw, please take one more sip for me, please..."

It soon became hard for me to avoid facing the unavoidable when I began having trouble convincing her to drink more than a sip or two. She got so weak she couldn't hold her head up or even sit up in her wheelchair. It tore me up to see her like this, but I didn't let it deter me. I continued my visits and stopped by every chance I could to check on her. She was usually asleep. Sometimes, I'd check with the nurses to see how she was and leave. Other times, I would sit quietly by her bed, wanting nothing more than to be near her. On many of those visits, I would feel my eyes welling up with tears and I fought it down, taking deep breaths, pacing around the room until I got myself under control again. It was difficult keeping my emotions in check, and there were many times I'd rush out of the room, speed-walk down the hall and out the front door to my car. I could usually sit beside her, staring upward and breathing deeply, in and out, until I could rein everything in. I don't know why it was so important to me as a young man to keep my emotions in check, but it was. I never cried over anything. This was my Mamaw, for goodness sake, and yet I foolishly thought I wasn't going to let her passing make me cry.

It was clear, by this time, that she wasn't going to be with us much longer. I felt driven to be with her when the time came. I didn't want my mamaw being alone when Jesus called her home. It was silly and selfish of me. She was going to be leaving for a better place, and whether anybody was with her or not wasn't going to

84

change this. Jesus had a place prepared for her and He was starting to call her to it. She had over ninety years of life. If anybody deserved to depart and be with the Lord, it was Mamaw. But now that I was faced with losing her, I didn't want to let her go.

I became obsessed with being by her side when she did leave and made countless trips to the nursing home each day. I was terrified every time the phone rang at home each night. I was certain that it would be the nursing home calling with the news that she was gone and I hadn't been with her. Sleep played a vicious game of tag with me each night, forcing me awake repeatedly, taunting me with dreams of the phone ringing. Morning finally came and I would quickly shower and race to the nursing home to see her.

On Tuesday, August 27, 2002, I had made several trips to check on her. Late that afternoon at work, I started inputting the daily sales reports from the previous week and all the invoices into the computer. When 5 PM rolled around, I closed my store, locked the door, and turned all the lights off but the one over the computer. I sat back down and finished the inputting. I knew I didn't have to rush to the nursing home because it had only been a few hours since my last trip to see her. I completed the little amount of work I had in about thirty minutes. I then locked everything up before heading to the nursing home.

I entered by the front entrance and walked straight ahead, down the hall past her old room to the end of the hall. I turned left, walked down a few doors, and entered her room. The curtains were pulled closed around her bed. I grabbed ahold of them and flung them open with a cheerful greeting ready for her. I never got the greeting out. I stood frozen in place, stunned and in shock. My dear, sweet Mamaw was lying in her bed, eyes gazing upward at nothing, her mouth frozen open in a ghastly expression. She was dressed but uncovered, lying there with one arm bent at the elbow and her hand raised upwards, permanently locked in some unknown gesture.

I moved to the chair by her bed, knees suddenly growing weak, and plopped down in it. Still in shock and at the mercy of gravity, my seated body continued its descent forward. I placed my elbows on my knees in time to catch my heavy head in my hands. I quietly moaned two words: "Oh, Mamaw…"

I don't know how long I sat next to her, holding my head in my hands, emotionless. I just stared at the floor, too numb to cry. My eyes remained dry the whole time. I am sure I was in shock because I have no recollection of any thoughts going through my stunned mind after entering her room. I simply sat beside her with my head down. I pulled myself to my feet and stumbled to my car. I drove back to my store and went inside to use the phone and let everyone in my family know that Mamaw was gone.

She had managed to stay with us another year from the time of her diagnosis of cancer.

First, I had to get word to Mom. She was still in Jamaica on her mission trip. She was prepared for this and had left me the phone number for the pastor in charge of her mission. Calling him and having to ask him to give this news to her was one of the most difficult things I have ever done. Or so I thought. It turns out there was a more challenging task for me to deal with, coming up soon enough.

Chapter 11
Road Trip Down Memory Lane

Mom had arranged for Mamaw to be transported to a funeral home in New Castle. She had taken care of everything before she left for Jamaica, so I didn't have to worry about anything, which was good. I withdrew into myself and don't remember much that happened after walking into Mamaw's room and finding she had passed away. I'm sure part of this was shock, but mostly, I think it was because of the guilt I was feeling. I shouldn't have been so overcome with guilt, but I was. I don't know why I felt like I should have been by her side that evening, but I did. I knew I would have been with her had I not stayed after work to input those papers. It bothered me that she was all alone when she died, and I couldn't get over the guilt I felt. It consumed me. She had always been a big part of my whole life. I had no memories of any time in my life that Mamaw hadn't been part of it. I felt like I had let her down because I wasn't there for her at the end and it was eating me up.

The funeral home sent a hearse later that night and transported Mamaw back to New Castle. I worked the next day, but have absolutely no recollection of the entire day until I got a call from Mom. The nursing home had forgotten to send Mamaw's dentures with her to the funeral home. I needed to drive them to New Castle and deliver them to the funeral home that evening so they could have her ready in time for the viewing.

I went to the nursing home to pick up her teeth. As I walked down the hall by her former room, every one of the nurses in that wing stopped me, gave me a hug, and told me how sorry they were. Some even cried. Mamaw had touched all their lives when they took care of her and they had cared about her. They shared in our loss. I rounded the corner and went to the nurse's station for the full-care wing and picked up a small brown lunch bag that had her teeth inside it. I carried the bag to my car, placed it on the passenger seat, and left for New Castle.

Mom was ten years old when Mamaw was in a bad car wreck. The wreck messed her teeth up badly. Mamaw did not like the way they looked and decided to have them all pulled out so she could get dentures. She didn't have many choices about how it was done back then. All her teeth were pulled out at the same time. She then had to go about a month with no teeth until all the swelling subsided. The dentist then fitted her with false teeth. She never took her teeth out except to brush them because she didn't want to be seen without her teeth. She even slept with them in. She had to have her teeth for her final public appearance.

It was a long, quiet drive for me as I brought Mamaw's teeth to her. I can look back on it now and see the humor in this. I can't imagine to many people can say they had to deliver a set of false teeth to a funeral home. Mamaw would surely have laughed at this, had she been there to see it. "Oh, Bobby," she would have said, as she chuckled and patted my knee. "I can't believe I left without my teeth!" and she would have laughed even more. That was the thing about Mamaw; she was always willing to laugh at herself. She was constantly saying or doing something silly, and when we laughed at her, she would be laughing right along with us. When she was done laughing, she would say, "Oh mercy," or, "Mercy me," and have everyone laughing again.

Unfortunately, I didn't see the humor in the situation that evening. As I made my way across the state in eerie silence, my eyes were constantly drawn to that brown bag sitting next to me. I still hadn't forgiven myself for working late the previous night, and the sight of that bag was a continuous reminder to me of my perceived negligence. As far as I was concerned, I had let my Mamaw down, and I couldn't stop thinking about this with her teeth next to me. I didn't think I would ever get to New Castle. The guilt was so strong that I still wasn't experiencing any feelings of grief. I was completely numb and oblivious to everything but my guilt.

Making it to the funeral home, I pulled into the parking lot and found a parking place near the front and pulled in. I jumped out of the van, bag in hand, and made my way inside, heading straight to the office. I told them who I was, handed them the bag of teeth, and made my way back to the van. I was in and out so quickly they were probably scratching their heads, wondering what had just happened. The brown bag with the teeth in it the only proof I had even been there. I didn't mean to be rude; that's not who I am. I was struggling internally with my own demons that evening, and I didn't want to be in the funeral home any longer than I had to be.

I decided to take myself on a trip down memory lane while I was in town, thinking it might help snap me out of the guilty state of mind I was struggling with. I took the highway into town and turned right on Riley Road. I took it east all the way across town to 14th Street, where I turned left. I drove a few blocks and turned left again into the neighborhood that had been the stomping grounds of my youth. I continued forward slowly, with the apartment complex on my left and the open fields of Sunnyside Elementary School on my right. I planned to take the first road left once I came to the last apartment building, but decided to pull off the road instead.

The apartment complex was on my left and had a courtyard in the center with a swimming pool. The first thing that came to mind when I saw the pool was that I had never swam in it. The entire time I lived across the street from it, I never did. It's funny how the mind can conjure up insignificant thoughts like that for no reason. The apartments also reminded me of another trivial memory from my time as a paperboy in 1972 and 1973. I delivered the *Indianapolis Star*, a morning paper. My route covered the entire housing addition and included the apartments. The sight of those buildings brought back all the funky odors I used to encounter in each foyer. Each building had a foyer on each end that accessed four units – two on the first floor, and two on the top. Each foyer had its own unique smell, for some reason, and none of them were pleasant. This was the easiest part of the route because I only had to step into each foyer and throw the rolled paper at each door. The odors weren't as noticeable then. It was each Friday and Saturday, when I had to knock on every customer's door to collect, that I couldn't avoid the stinky aromas.

I delivered papers for a year. I could deliver them on my bike when the weather was nice. I'd get up at the crack of dawn and roll each newspaper and slide a rubber band on it. I had a newspaper bag that slipped over my head like a poncho, with a large pouch in the front and the back. The amount of papers I delivered were tightly squeezed into both sides of the bag. It was so full and heavy that I couldn't lift it over my head. I had to push the sides as far apart as I could on the floor and crawl in between them on my belly. I then slid my head through the hole and struggled to a position on all fours, like a dog. From here, using my hands and knees, I would push the bag up until I could get both feet flat on the floor. Like a weightlifter doing squats with a barbell, I would heave myself up and into a standing position with the bag's weight resting on my scrawny little shoulders. For my next trick, I had to find the perfect balance of weight with the overstuffed bag and my bike. That wasn't the hard part. Maintaining this balance while I pedaled down the road, throwing papers at front porches, was the real tricky part.

This reminded me of the morning I got chased by a dog in the middle of my balancing act. I was three roads over from my house, and still carrying a pretty full load. Out of nowhere, a Doberman came barreling down the road at me, barking like he was going to eat me for breakfast. I did what any brave young boy would do: I pedaled like there was no tomorrow, convinced I had a real chance of outrunning the beast behind me. I made a turn towards the sidewalk at the same time the owner hollered for the dog. In perfect unison, the dog turned and hightailed it home as I went flying over the handlebars. Newspapers were flying everywhere as I did a perfect somersault on my way to the ground. Thank goodness it was grass I was heading for – or so I thought. It turned out, my landing wasn't so perfect. I hit the ground hard, sliding forward from my momentum. I was pedaling a hundred miles an hour, after all. My body came to a stop. I was stung by a bee before I could suck the air back into my lungs. I had picked up a passenger in my pant leg during my slide. One that wasn't very happy for the free ride and he took it out on my leg. In avoiding the dog bite, I had been rewarded with a bee-sting. This was nothing compared to delivering newspapers in the winter. This was hard enough walking around in the deep snow. It was nearly impossible lugging that monstrous bag of newspapers through it.

Returning to reality, I looked away from the apartments. To my immediate right was where the old baseball backstop fence had been. This was the location of countless pick-up baseball games I played in as a kid. Every week during the summer, kids from all around the area would meet at this decrepit ball diamond for a game. Sides would be picked and then a bat tossed and caught by one of the captains with one hand. The other captain would place his hand on top of his hand. They would alternate hands to the top of the bat, and whoever's hand covered the knob on the top of the bat won the toss. This meant he got to pick whether his team would take the field or bat first. If we were short players, then right field would be designated out of bounds. If someone hit the ball over there, they were automatically out. We played fast pitch without wearing any protective gear – not even batting helmets. If anybody got beaned in the head by a pitch, they had to pick themselves up, brush off the dust, and choke back any sign of tears if they knew what was good for them. We were all Cincinnati Reds fans and tried to act like our favorite player. This would have been from 1973 to 1976 when the Big Red Machine was the best team in the world.

Across the field stood Sunnyside Elementary School, and it looked the same as it did when I attended it in the sixties. I had gone there twice: for kindergarten, when we lived with Mamaw for half a year, and for third through sixth grade when I lived in the neighborhood. I was amazed at how little it had changed on the outside. I could see the basketball court I played on at recess during the school year and on many summer days. I could see, in my mind's eye, the home plate painted on the ground next to the building and the strike zone painted on the wall. I spent countless hours throwing a rubber ball at that wall, perfecting my fastball. Thanks to that wall, I had quite the fastball in my pitching arsenal. Just ask any of the guys I hit with it in Little League.

I put the car in drive and made the left turn, drove a block around the apartment complex, and made another left on Plymouth Street. I pulled off the road in front of the second house on the right. This was the house I grew up in during those four years I went to Sunnyside. It was hard to believe this little house had four bedrooms. It looked exactly the way I remembered it. Even the color was the same. This little excursion was like going back in time. The open lot next to the house was no longer there. Instead, the lot now had two houses on it.

Mamaw visited us quite often when we lived here. She would come over to make a pot of chili, bring her homemade chicken pot pie, or some other dish for supper. She would do this so Mom wouldn't have to cook when she got home. Sitting at the end of my old driveway, I remembered one time, Mom had to be out of town for some reason, and Mamaw stayed with us. We talked her into taking us to Top Hat Pizza on Broad Street, clear on the other side of town. We couldn't all fit in her car, so she had to drive our family car. It was a red Opel station wagon with a stick shift. I don't think Mamaw had driven a stick shift for a long time. Watching her try to drive that giant station wagon with a stick shift was hilarious. Grinding through the gears as she struggled to work the clutch and shift gears simultaneously was quite an adventure. Of course, I was sitting in the backseat, trying desperately to keep from laughing too loudly.

The Opel was made and imported from Germany. This road trip to Top Hat with five kids happened in the late fall, so the temperature was dropping quite a bit when we all climbed into the car. Mamaw managed to get us all to the restaurant in one piece without destroying the transmission. We went inside to enjoy the best pizza anywhere. Little did we know, the ride there wasn't the real adventure at all. It turned out to be the opening act for the night.

It was dark and raining by the time we finished our pizza and went outside. Not only that, but the temperature was dropping and freezing the rain on the windshield. We had no idea how to turn on the lights, the heater, the windshield defrosters, or the windshield wipers. All the controls on the dashboard were written in German. We were quite the sight, sitting in that parking lot. Mamaw was behind the steering wheel. I was in the passenger seat and my four brothers and sisters were in the back. We were all trying to figure out how to read the controls. Mamaw would try one button and the flashers would go on. She'd say, "Oh, mercy, that's not it," and we would all bust out laughing. She'd reach for another knob and accidentally hit the horn, scaring us. This was followed by another round of laughter. At last, through the process of elimination, she figured out where the right controls were. With a sketchy knowledge of where everything she needed was, she could drive us home. We were all so tickled over the whole spectacle we laughed the whole way home.

The Plymouth Street house was only about eight blocks from Mamaw's house. I used to ride my bike over to visit her whenever I could. This was where we lived when I'd go sit with her to listen to the Trojans game. I would ride over to mow her yard every week or for no other reason than to surprise her. I played little league baseball over by Bakers Park and would ride my bike to many games. If she couldn't make it to my games, I would stop by her house on my way home to see her.

My next stop on the memory train was those eight blocks to her house. I drove back out to 14th Street, turned left, and drove past

Sunnyside on the left. A little further was Jack's Donuts on the right. I could almost taste those amazing donuts as I drove by. When I had my paper route, I liked to get up early and ride my bike to Jack's first. You haven't lived until you've eaten warm glazed yeast donuts fresh out of the fryer. Next to Jack's Donuts, and in the same building, was Mary's. This was a tiny diner-type restaurant where the food was decent enough but nothing special. Mamaw would bring me here occasionally because it was the only place in town that served cow's tongue. This is the most disgusting food I have ever heard of, and it looked as nasty as it sounded. But Mamaw loved eating cow's tongue. I suspect she developed a taste for this from growing up during the Great Depression. I am sure families had to eat every part of the animals they raised or go hungry.

Right past Jack's was the Dairy Queen we used to walk to from her house, where we'd get Peanut Buster Parfaits and Dilly Bars. At 14th and O Street was Tony's Pizza on the right, and Mamaw's house was two houses down on the left. Behind Tony's Pizza was Bonnie's, the little beauty shop that took care of Mamaw's hair for most of her life. I turned left on O Street, and behind the first house, I turned right going up the alley that led behind Mamaw's house to see the back yard. The first thing I saw was that the new owners had cut down her beautiful maple tree in the backyard. That thing was huge and shaded the entire backyard. It had one limb that had a rope swing that each one of us kids had swung on thousands of times. But it was gone. Then I could see that her little white shed next to the alley was gone too. Otherwise, the house looked the same, and so did the neighborhood. But it wasn't. It never would be to me, no matter how many times I drove by it in the future. It would always be Mamaw's house, no matter how it looked.

We lived with her for about six months when I was in half-day kindergarten, around 1968 or so. I can recall some of my time at her house then. I remember her driving me to school and running out of the car to join the kids at recess. Mamaw liked to tell people how she would drop me off and all the girls would chase me around the parking lot. I don't remember that part. I do remember I had to bring a floor rug and keep it in a barrel with the other kids' rugs. I would have to get it out and unroll it on the floor for naptime each day. It's funny what the brain chooses to remember. The missing tree in her backyard made me sad but, overall, the sight of her house overwhelmed me with good memories and brought a smile to my face. I could still see her coming out her back door with a cup of lemonade for me. The cup was one of those colored aluminum types that dripped water as the cold cup met the warm air. Lemonade always tasted better in those cups.

Sitting in her alley, I recalled all those wonderful times at Dewart Lake. Swimming in the lake and how excited we'd all get on those rare occasions when Mamaw would join us. She had this blue one-piece suit that was very modest, and she always wore a bathing cap to keep her hair dry. The countless games she played with us, just her and a bunch of kids, or a mixture of kids and adults. She was so animated when she talked, with her hands and arms flapping all around while she spoke. One time, we all got real tickled about how she moved her arms and hands when she talked and we were all laughing about it, including Mamaw. Then Marta said, "Aunt Thelma, can you talk without moving your arms?"

Mamaw said, "Well, I suppose I can."

To find out, Marta loosely held Mamaw's arms to her sides. It was like she had cut off her brain from her mouth. Mamaw sat there, babbling, unable to form words. She'd try but kept pausing, as she couldn't seem to get the words out. It was the funniest thing I ever saw. Marta only held her arms a few minutes and mercifully released her arms. Mamaw laughed with the rest of us. She made the comment that she couldn't talk, no matter how hard she tried, which sent us all into another bout of laughter.

I glanced at the spot next to the missing shed and recalled the large stalks and leaves of rhubarb that grew there every summer. My friends liked to break off a stalk and sprinkle salt on it to eat it raw. My family loved it when Mamaw made her rhubarb pie every summer. Everyone but me, that is. I was never a fan of rhubarb.

From here, I headed north on 14th to Grand Avenue. We had lived in a duplex home near the end of the street. It was next to the Nazarene church that my Uncle George had helped build, and which he attended every Sunday. Marta and her husband, Rusty, were married at this church and I was a candle lighter in the wedding – brown leisure suit and all. The house we lived in next door was gone. I think the church bought it and tore it down, but I'm not sure of this in totality. Unbeknownst to me at the time, I would be back here in two days. Marta's church family had volunteered to prepare a meal for us after Mamaw's services. I drove past the vacant lot our house used to sit on and worked my way back north, past the seventh-grade building I attended, over to Broad Street, turning right.

I passed Top Hat Pizza and couldn't help but smile as thoughts of that night in the red Opel returned. A little past this on the right was the small white house we had moved to from Plymouth Street. I thought about how small the house was. It was a two-bedroom house with one bathroom for Mom and five kids. Mom had the main bedroom, and Laura and Amy shared the other. My brothers and I slept in the attic. They weren't really bedrooms we slept in. The attic had one large room when you entered, which Scott and James shared. I had the small room in the back to myself, a benefit to being the oldest. The floors weren't carpeted, but we didn't care. The house was very modest, and sleeping in the attic sounds worse than it was. To three young boys, it was like sleeping in a clubhouse every night. At the end of the block was a Burger Chef.

We didn't have much money back then. Raising five kids didn't leave much extra money for Mom, so we rarely ate out. The thing about growing up poor is that we never considered ourselves to be poor. This is a strong testament to my mother and the way she raised all five of us. I didn't miss eating out or designer clothes because I wasn't used to them anyway. When I did do something special, like eating out, it was a real treat and I appreciated it a whole lot more when it did happen. Those meals after church with Mamaw were about the only times I ate out during the fall, winter, and spring. In the summer, she always stopped on the way to the lakes, and on the way home, and that was also special to me. I wasn't used to eating out, so it didn't matter that it didn't happen very often. Then we moved next to a Burger Chef. Back then, they would sometimes run hamburgers four for a dollar. This was huge for me and my brothers and sisters because now Mom could afford to leave us a few bucks to walk over to Burger Chef for supper. They had this topping bar, so I could pile all the toppings I wanted on one burger and fill myself up. Mom would treat us to burger nights quite a bit, and Mamaw would take us occasionally as well. Burger Chef was later bought out by Hardee's a long time ago, so it was a Hardee's now.

I pulled into their parking lot, turned around, and headed west on Broad Street. I had one more stop on the Mamaw memory tour before heading home. I wanted to drive around the *Courier Times* and feel her memories from there. I drove by the front and it looked the same. I then went to the parking lot in the rear of the building, and even that looked unchanged. I could see my bike leaning against the wall while I walked through that back door to surprise Mamaw. I knew the inside would look foreign to me. All the typesetting machines would be gone, and the area was now occupied by a bunch of cubicles and computers. But sitting alone in my van, looking at this building that seemed frozen in time, I was flooded with the most memories of Mamaw. For the first time since losing her, I felt the pangs of this loss and my eyes filled with tears. I took big, deep breaths and turned up the radio for a distraction while I fought to regain control of myself. That trip down memory lane was nice and had stirred up many wonderful memories of Mamaw. That final stop at her work had been too much, though, and had brought me back down to the reality that she was gone.

I got back on the road and headed back to Bedford. By this time, it was dark outside and I drove home in complete silence. I was alone in my dark van with my thoughts deep in some dark place I hadn't realized I had created. Before I knew it, I was home. I kissed my wife and went straight to my recliner, still residing somewhere in my head, struggling with my turmoil over Mamaw's death.

Chapter 12
Saying Goodbye

    The next day was Mamaw's scheduled viewing and visitation at the funeral home. I continued to be stuck deep in my own thoughts, buried somewhere inside myself as I went through the motions of preparing for the drive back to New Castle in a zombie-like state. I was still struggling with the guilt of letting her down by not being by her side. My heart was broken from the thoughts of her dying alone. I was so ashamed of myself for choosing to work late over being on time to the nursing home. I felt like I had let my mom down as well. I can deal with anything, but I couldn't bear the thought that I had disappointed my mother. Logic had disappeared for me with Mamaw's passing because I knew my mother would never blame me for this. But, I couldn't seem to stop the guilty feelings that were overwhelming me. I continued to languish in this hell I had created for myself all that day.

    Mom had reserved rooms for us at the Steve Alford Inn, which was a short distance from the funeral home. This meant I had to pack overnight bags for the trip. I picked out the dark suit I wanted to wear and then had Bobby and Robby try on different jackets, dress pants, and dress shirts until I found the ones that looked presentable on them. I was a lot bigger than they were. This made it a challenging task trying to find something that didn't dwarf them. I didn't want them looking like they were playing dress-up. I found dress clothes that would suffice. I let them pick out ties to wear.

    The time had come to leave, and I loaded the van and departed for New Castle. I drove, but have absolutely no memory of the three-hour trip. I arrived at the hotel and checked into my two rooms. Once the kids were settled into their room, I went to mine to try and relax until it was time for the viewing. Relaxing wasn't going to happen for me, no matter how tired I was. I somehow managed to survive the wait and got ready to depart for the funeral home. The five of us grandkids and our families met Mom at the funeral home about fifteen minutes before the viewing was scheduled to begin.

    People started arriving right after I had gotten there, so I forced down the inner turmoil I was struggling with and slipped into hotel manager mode. I greeted everyone that came into the viewing room as soon as they arrived. Most of them were family members I hadn't seen in years. For the next few hours, I hugged and visited with loved ones and long forgotten friends, and shared many stories about Mamaw. Every story was usually funny and I inevitably ended up laughing about each one. It was exactly as Mamaw would have wanted the evening to go.

I wouldn't go so far as to say this was therapeutic for me. Nor did it help me deal with the demon's I was facing with my loss. I'm sure the visiting and laughing helped many people, but for me, it only helped get me through the evening. After the last person left, I was finally able to drop out of hotel manager mode. I was one of the best when it came to putting on this persona while running a hotel and dealing with other people. I could bury all emotions and control my reactions in any situation – even at the funeral of my beloved Mamaw, it seemed. By all outward appearances, hotel manager mode allowed me to be the perfect host: confident, friendly, and carefree while interacting with others.

When it was over, I was drained from the hours I had spent playing the good son and grandson. I returned to the hotel and collapsed, mentally and physically, until the next morning's final viewing and burial. For me, as soon as I got undressed, I became a zombie: numb and unaware of everything around me. After playing the good host at the viewing, I simply didn't have anything left in my tank. I spent the rest of the evening in a vegetative state, staring at the television without watching it. I felt hollow and dead inside. The nearest restaurant was a truck stop about a mile away. I'm told we all met for dinner there that evening, but I have no memory of this. I've heard many times that the brain will sometimes bury traumatic memories. The grief and guilt I struggled with that day must have been a fierce battle if I've forgotten so many entire events.

The next morning arrived and I was filled with dread. I knew that Mamaw had already departed and was with the Lord. I couldn't help this feeling of a finality approaching, like a runaway freight train that I had no control over. Mamaw was gone and there wasn't anything that could fill the hole in my heart without her. Like my mother, she had always been a part of my life. Once this day was over, I would have to face a life with no Mamaw. This added to the

98

internal struggle I was dealing with, over my guilt for not being with her when she departed. I kept pushing these emotions down, rather than facing them. I thought I was supposed to be strong for my mom and siblings, and my own family. I was the oldest child and a husband and father. I needed to be the pillar of strength for everyone, particularly my mom. She had lost her mother, and this crushed me more than everything else. I loved my mamaw, but I cherish my mom dearly and cannot imagine losing her. Just thinking about this causes me to tear up at once. Shoot, I can't think about losing my mom at any time without getting emotional. It broke my heart when I thought about what she was going through during Mamaw's services. I pushed these thoughts down with everything else.

I returned to the funeral home and slipped back into hotel manager mode for the final visitation and the upcoming service. My heart was too heavy this day to socialize much, and I ended up avoiding conversations and personal contact as much as I could. I spent most of my time at the rear of the room, as far from Mamaw as I could get, avoiding even looking toward her. At one point, I had to sneak out the back door and walk the parking lot for a few minutes. I paced back and forth, huffing and puffing like I was in labor, trying to fight back the tears that wanted to break out from behind the walls I had built. I managed to push these emotions back down and got myself under control again. I went back inside and returned to the back of the room. Mom came back, at some point, and told me it was time for the service to begin.

Marsha and I moved to the front of the room and took our seats in the front row with the rest of my family. Mom wanted to conduct the services at the funeral home, which was the right decision. No minister could honor Mamaw more than the daughter that was the light of her life. She started the services by thanking everyone for coming to say goodbye to her mom. She then stepped aside while a few family members performed special tributes to Mamaw. My niece, Hannah, played her flute and her sister, Taylor, read a poem she had written about Mamaw. My baby sister, Amy, with that beautiful voice of hers, sang an amazing song that touched the hearts of everyone. Mom had everybody gathered join her in singing Mamaw's favorite hymn, "How Great Thou Art."

I am sure this was Mamaw's favorite song. I remember many times as a child listening to her sing along as it played over her little radio. I'm not sure how often she had cleaning day, but it was once a month. This spring-type cleaning occurred on a Sunday after church. She would turn her little AM radio to a station playing church music while she cleaned. When this song came on, she would stop whatever she was doing and sing along. I am certain she was watching over us that day, singing this beautiful song one final time with us. I could hear her voice lifted with us.

These thoughts made the wall I had built inside crack slightly. My eyes began to fill with tears so I shifted my gaze up toward the ceiling, struggling to calm myself down. At the end of the song, I felt like I had myself under control again. Mom began her sermon about Mamaw. I turned my gaze toward her so I could concentrate completely as she spoke her personal tribute to Mamaw's life.

As soon as she began to speak, my gaze caught sight of Mamaw lying next to Mom in her casket, and I lost all control. I began moaning softly but it quickly grew in volume until I was moaning loud enough for everyone to hear me. I cried out, "Oh, Mamaw," and began sobbing uncontrollably. Crying would be describing it too mildly and doesn't do justice to what I did. I wailed. I was so overcome by everything I had been struggling with since the night of her passing – the guilt, sorrow, concern for Mom, and everything else I had pushed deep within me. It all had become too much for me to control. I could no longer contain the pressure of it all twisting and turning inside me when I saw her lying so solemnly. Suddenly, there was no hiding from it any longer. Mamaw was gone. The reality of my loss hit me hard, breaking through my walls, and everything I was holding inside came busting out. Once I saw her tiny body lying in that casket, I was done. There was no calling it back, so deep was my sorrow.

I sobbed like a little baby for a bit, then I'd loudly moan again, "Oh, Mamaw," and let out a wail that had to be heart-wrenching to hear. I released a sound I didn't know could come from a human being: a long, loud cry – almost a howl, filled with my grief. I felt Marsha put her hand on my back, rubbing and patting me in an attempt to comfort me. But my grief was too deep, and there was no consoling me.

I would sob and whimper for a few minutes before being overcome again with my sorrow. I released another animalistic howl of grief that ripped my heart wide open for my mamaw. My poor mother was surely struggling to control her own grief. She had to continue with her message to the gathering over the sounds of my suffering right in front of her. I'm sure my wails, filled with my grief and broken heart, touched everyone. How could the depths of my sorrow not touch them as it burst forth, uncontrollably, in front of them? The raw emotions coming from me had to be felt across that room. I'm sure it caused many of the women to start crying, and more than a few men stared at the ceiling with their own tear-filled eyes, struggling to keep themselves in check. These people knew me, and it had to be tough on them to hear Mamaw's big, hulking grandson bawling his eyes out in front of them. I didn't turn around and check. I was too lost in my grief to even care what was happening around me. My total meltdown with grief was like the Old Testament mourners. They would become so overcome from the death of a loved one that they tore their clothing and fell to their knees crying.

I was so engulfed in my grief that I was, on all accounts, oblivious to anything else. I didn't hear a word of Mom's sermon; at least, I can't recall any of it. I'm not sure how she was even able to deliver it with my anguish unfolding a few feet in front of her. I don't know how she could remain in control and keep from crying herself, seeing her firstborn child losing all self-control right before her eyes. She was crying with me. The truth is, I don't know how my grief affected anyone. I was a lost soul during Mamaw's services that day, totally consumed with agony and despair.

I didn't fight it. I couldn't. My heart was ripped open, and the pain of losing Mamaw was more than I could handle. I had fallen into the abyss her death had created in me. I was drowning in my sorrow and I didn't care who witnessed it. I couldn't have stopped it, anyway. Once my wall crumbled, it was like a dam had busted and I didn't have the tools to stop the onslaught. I was a prisoner to its release and had no choice but to let it run its course. And run its course it did, through the whole service. I sat there with my chest torn wide open, as my pain and anguish filled the entire room. It fed the sadness already present like gasoline thrown on a fire, and I am certain there couldn't have been many people who weren't affected by my suffering. This deep sorrow is contagious, like a yawn in public that takes on a life of its own as it spreads from person to person.

Mom finished this eulogy of Mamaw with a prayer. I calmed down a little and wasn't squalling uncontrollably by the time she got to the Amen. I stood with my mom and my siblings, and we moved to the foot of the casket. We lined up for the procession of people to come forward and express their condolences and spend a final moment with Mamaw. I may have kept the wailing from escaping, but there was no chance of stopping the steady flow of tears. Everyone had just witnessed my outpouring of grief, and many of them wanted to hug me and whisper words of encouragement in my ear as a sign of support for me and my bereavement. The tears flowed unashamedly down my cheeks as I thanked each one while returning their hugs.

As my relatives approached, I could see the sympathy they felt for my suffering and the anguish in their eyes. Many were still shedding tears of their own as they approached me. The sight of this went straight to my broken heart and sent me into another round of sobbing as we held and comforted each other.

A lot of people were at Mamaw's service. Everyone loved her. She was ninety years old, and most of her friends of days-gone-by had already passed away. She had impacted so many lives with her kindness and sincerity. This caused many younger generations to feel the need to pay their respects. The endless line of people worked its way past Mamaw's casket. I quietly let out a sigh of relief, exhausted from the emotional breakdown and all the crying.

I remained in place as my whole family came forward and took turns hugging me. Not a word was spoken as each member held me in their arms. None were needed. This simple gesture let me know they were all there for me and always would be. This helped me regain my composure. When I had received the final hug, we all exited the room so they could prepare Mamaw for the ride to her grave. She was going to lie next to the love of her life, after losing him so many years ago.

Mom had all five of Mamaw's grandkids, plus Bobby and Robby, and herself as pallbearers. We moved to the rear entrance and waited for the staff to bring Mamaw to us. I don't know if I could control myself at this point or if my body was dehydrated from all the tears, but I finally stopped crying. I remained in control of myself when the funeral home staff brought her out. I managed to do my part in loading her casket into the hearse without incident. I walked toward the front of the vehicle procession, where Marsha and my family were waiting for me. I always drove, but Marsha knew I was in no condition to be driving for this trip, so she was in the driver's seat when I arrived, God love her thoughtful heart. The short ride to the cemetery was made in complete silence. I am certain Marsha and the kids were in shock themselves. They had always seen me as a strong person who was always in control and to witness my meltdown had left them speechless. I'm sure they were worried about me, but couldn't find any words of comfort to give me. What could they say? Marsha kept reaching over and patting me on the arm or leg and asking if I was all right. I could see the concern in her eyes as well.

I was exhausted by this time, and the trip to the cemetery remains a blur in my mind. I vaguely recall walking over to the hearse and carrying Mamaw to the gravesite. I remember walking to the front row of chairs that were designated for family and taking my place with my mom and siblings. I thought the worst of my inner turmoil had passed. I didn't think anything could be left after my outburst and breakdown at the funeral home. I was convinced I had gotten myself under control and could make it through the short graveside service.

I was wrong. As soon as my cousin Bryan opened his mouth to begin the service, I lost it again. I sat there sobbing uncontrollably through the entire graveside service. I didn't wail, but I do remember a few loud moans of, "Oh, Mamaw," that escaped from my mouth while my grief poured out anew. Bryan finished his sermon, and I calmed myself down as he said the final prayer of the service. I went back to my van and climbed into the passenger seat once again. The next stop was at the Nazarene Church where the ladies of the church had prepared a meal for a final family gathering.

Marsha drove. I remember that much. I seriously doubt I could have. We got to the church and I went inside and removed my jacket and tie. I was completely drained from all the raw emotion that Mamaw's funeral had pulled from me. When I sat down, I felt like I was done crying. The reception was like our family reunions of the past combined, with everyone there coming from all the different branches of my family tree. That's how loved Mamaw was. Even my dad and his wife Ginger came to the reception. They had been to the services, but I hadn't spent any time with them, so I sat with them at the reception. Everyone seemed to find their way to show me their sympathy and support once again, because of my meltdown. I got more hugs and words of encouragement. I could finally talk about Mamaw without getting choked up, so I'm sure this made everyone feel better about my well-being.

The real test was yet to come. Amy had put together a tribute to Mamaw, and I was certain I wouldn't be able to make it through that in one piece. After everyone had eaten, it was time to watch the video. Amy had done an amazing job putting together a slideshow of pictures from Mamaw's life. Most of the pictures were of us kids growing up, which didn't surprise me at all. We were all a huge part of Mamaw's life, from my birth in 1963 until her death in 2002. Sitting there, seeing these images of her life – and of *my* life – I could appreciate the beautiful tribute Amy had created without bawling my eyes out. As each of the images rotated on the screen, I could feel a smile forming. Mamaw had that effect on me.

Chapter 13
A Memory of Mamaw

My Aunt Thelma was an incredible person. She was a lady before her time, playing basketball and being a tomboy. She was always very positive and never had a negative comment about anything.

She always made everyone laugh when she would get so busy talking that her hands would be flying all over the place. Nothing was funnier than to see her get so absorbed in what she was saying that she'd end up hitting something, or someone, with those flailing arms. This must run in the family because my dad and myself both talk with our hands.

Aunt Thelma loved everybody and everybody loved her. I was always so excited to get to see her. I loved it when she called my dad "Buddy."

I remember the last time Aunt Thelma was at my house. It was for Thanksgiving and she was in the early stages of her dementia. Her daughter Sheryl brought her over and I remember her telling Aunt Thelma, "Mom, you won't know everybody so just enjoy the day." I think she did have a good time that day.

Aunt Thelma had a joyful laugh that was very contagious. Everyone who heard it ended up laughing along with her.

I was so very lucky to have this wonderful lady in my family.

Love and Prayers.

Marta J. (Solomon) Davis

Chapter 14
Enough is Enough

The story was supposed to end here. I have been blessed with a wonderful family and love my life. My lovely wife retired in 2012. I'm unable to work because of health issues so I get to spend every waking moment with her. Our three granddaughters are growing up and a real joy to be with. My life couldn't be better. The book was finished and titled *Memories of Mamaw; Losing a Loved One to Dementia.* I was very proud of the book and published it in October 2017. A week later, my world was rocked. My dear wife was diagnosed with dementia.

There were signs, of course. Trivial things on the surface that normally would have seemed insignificant. Forgetting where the car keys were. Misplacing her cell phone. A little alarm went off in my head with each occurrence. These signs aren't so insignificant when her father was lost to Alzheimer's. When it started happening more frequently in 2016, the little alarm was becoming hard to silence. I found myself spending a significant amount of time searching for the same misplaced items – car keys, cell phone, checkbook, and her glasses. It really scared me when it got to this point.

I never shared my concerns with her to keep her from worrying about it. I knew she would. She is a worrier, anyway. Had I told her I was worried, she would have immediately jumped to Alzheimer's as the cause. She had an appointment coming up with her doctor when the symptoms began worsening. I decided it would be best to give her doctor a heads-up. I stopped by his office a few days before her appointment. I told one of his nurses about everything going on and asked her to mention it to the doctor. I had hoped he would investigate it further when she was with him.

The day of the appointment rolled around. I asked Marsha to mention that she was constantly misplacing things to initiate a discussion. She came back from her appointment happy with the visit. She said he had told her misplacing things wasn't anything to be worried about. She mentioned her dad to him and was told she had no reason to be concerned about having Alzheimer's. He said her memory was fine. I was glad her mind was put at ease but I continued to be concerned.

Her misplacing things began happening with much more frequency over the next year. It got to where I would search for her phone a dozen times a day. Every day became an unending scavenger hunt for the various things she'd misplace throughout the day. That alarm had become a full-blown siren that couldn't be ignored.

Marsha has always been a nice dresser. She never went into public without looking her best in nice clothes and make-up. She's not someone you would ever run into at the grocery store wearing hair curlers and a bathrobe. This meant she always over-packed for every vacation or business trip we went on. We used to go to Las Vegas three times a year - our anniversary, the 4th of July, and in the fall. She attended every annual Hotel and Motel Association conference with me. We drove our kids to Florida for two weeks every Christmas for fifteen years or so. Every trip had one thing that I could always count on. Marsha would have two full-size suitcases, a carry-on size suitcase, and three or four handbags packed for each trip. She'd start packing two weeks out to make sure she didn't forget anything.

The two of us drove to the Blue Ridge Mountains Christian Writer's Conference in May 2015. She started packing for this trip six weeks in advance. I'd tell her she had plenty of time to pack. I would walk her through the calendar to help her understand. This went on for weeks. We'd be watching TV and she would get up to go to the bathroom and not come back. I'd go check on her and there she was, going through her clothes and packing. I let her work on her packing whenever she wanted to. I laid out two full-size suitcases and she got to work filling them up. They were full in no time. She then started worrying that she packed the wrong clothes. She spent hours each day trying clothes on and moving them back and forth from the suitcase and the closet. I tried to convince her it didn't matter what she took. She always looked good in whatever she wore. My words had no effect on her worries. In the end, I brought in another suitcase which she did not hesitate to fill up. This didn't solve anything because she kept trying outfits on as she packed and unpacked different ones. I packed my stuff the night before we left. It all fit into a small carry-on size suitcase. The next morning, I loaded the car with our bags. We have a Ford Fusion which is a small car but it has a huge trunk. The trunk was so full I could barely close it. We were only going to be gone from home for five days.

As mentioned earlier, there are several types of dementia. Most forms are the result of the death of brain cells. There is no cure for these dementias. My grandmother had a mini-stroke that killed a small amount of brain cells that led to more and more brain cells dying. This is known as vascular dementia. Marsha's dad had Alzheimer's that caused his dementia. This dementia is caused by a breakdown of the connection or bridge between brain cells. This breakdown slows the thinking process because the affected brain cells can no longer communicate. Enough of these connections break down and parts of the brain begin to shrink. This shrinking of the brain is known as atrophy and is irreversible. The affected brain cells die from the broken connections. The symptom for these damaged bridges between cells is slower brain function. It takes longer for a person to respond or react.

A CT Scan is done on the brain to look for any abnormalities. This test will also distinguish any atrophy. An electroencephalogram (EEG) is typically done to determine electrical activity. This test can determine if the brain cells are communicating. The connection between the cells is damaged or broken will cause an issue of slow or no electrical flow during the test. The EEG can usually determine the specific area of the brain if an issue exists.

This was the dreaded news we received for my dear wife in October. Her CT scan showed atrophy in both the left and right sides of her frontal lobe. The diagnosis from the radiologist was dementia. Her doctor wouldn't diagnose her with Alzheimer's, even with her family history. The EEG was done in January and confirmed that her brain took longer than normal to respond to the electrical stimuli of the test. Final diagnosis by the neurologist was dementia as well.

Early diagnosis of any illness is important. The earlier it is caught, the more likely it can be cured. There is no cure for dementia but early diagnosis is still important. The sooner you catch it, the more likely the medicines can slow its progress. The problem is that early detection of dementia isn't as simple as it sounds. As we age, a normal deterioration of brain cells can happen. This can lead to a natural occurrence of dementia. Therefore, many people tend to associate memory loss with aging and give no consideration of an underlying medical condition.

The worst problem for me was her well-meaning friends. Marsha and I began talking about her trouble remembering things. She was becoming aware that it was getting harder for her. She would talk with one of her friends or someone at church about it. She'd tell them how she was always losing her phone or the car keys. They would tell her it was nothing to be concerned with because they forget things too. This prevented me from being able to coax her into getting the proper testing without seeming to force it on her. I don't blame or fault any of them. They were unaware of the real situation we were facing. I stayed away from this topic for the time being.

It wasn't long before her forgetfulness got unmistakably worse. I was used to looking for her phone a dozen times a day. There was no denying a decline when I would have to find it fifteen minutes after the last search. She began misplacing more and more things at an alarming rate. Most of the time, I could find the phone, car keys, checkbooks, combs, debit card, and such in her purse. Whenever she would panic from losing something, I would always ask her to check her purse first. I began joking with her by telling her to look in her purse before panicking. I'd say, "Go look in your purse. Everything always ends up in there." She would laugh with me, especially when she found the item in her purse.

Things didn't always end up in her purse. She'd set things down and forget where she set them right away. I had begun keeping track of her movements out of fear. It scared me to death she might be searching for some misplaced item without my knowledge. I didn't want her getting all worked up if I could avoid it. I made it a point to help her search every time she misplaced something, at once, to keep her from panicking. I'd tell her to take a deep breath and relax, and then promise her we would find it, reminding her that we always did. Together, we would check her purse and then I would go to the last place I had seen her. We rarely had to tear the house apart to find anything. It was more about keeping her calm and proving to her that the item in question wasn't lost. In the long run, I got her to where panic wasn't her first reaction. She even began quoting me by saying that we always find it.

It is so important to reassure your loved ones during this early stage of the disease. The more worked up they get, the more inept and useless they feel. Nobody should feel this way. Especially, those in the initial stages of dementia. It's not easy to exercise patience under normal circumstances. It's hard the fifteenth time you're looking for a cell phone. You must force yourself to always exercise patience. If finding their phone is important to them, then it should be important to you. Telling them not to worry about it, or it'll show up, doesn't help at all. You might as well be talking to a wall. Finding a lost item will become a fixation for them. Drop whatever you're doing and find the item. Be sure to include them in your search. Chances are, they're going to follow you around anyway.

We both maintained separate checking accounts. We'd done this since we were married. We split up the monthly household expenses giving us both certain bills we were responsible for paying. We paid our own credit cards and shared in the discretionary spending. She stopped paying her bills at some point early that summer. I didn't catch this until the collection agencies started sending bills. I took over all the bill paying from then on. She no longer needs to worry about bills and I no longer find myself hunting down her checkbook.

I asked her one day to drive to the ATM and withdraw some money from my bank account. She looked at me like I had asked her to fly to the moon. I repeated what I wanted her to do and she informed me she wasn't sure how to do it. I explained to her step-by-step how to use the ATM and I wrote down the pin number for her. While she was getting ready, she came to me three or four times. She would apologize before asking me to explain what she had to do again. I told her not to worry about it, I'd write it all down for her. She approached me one more time before she left and asked if we could go over the notes one more time. I explained it again and then told her not to worry about it if she had trouble. It was no big deal. We could get it later if we had to.

She was gone much longer than expected and I began to worry. I always worry about her getting lost when she leaves, even though she hadn't shown any signs of this. Sometime later, she would come home and hand me a bank envelope with the money in it. She told me she couldn't get the ATM to work. She said she kept trying but had to go inside the bank. I told her that didn't matter and that she had done well. I gave her a hug and a kiss and thanked her. The smile on her face assured me she wasn't going to worry over this.

One day, she started realizing the change in her memory. I could sense the frustration when she misplaced something. It was hard for her to ignore when it would happen shortly after we had just found the item. I eased her stress with our check the purse routine. She'd follow this with, "I know, it'll show up. It always does" and we'd laugh together. I casually mentioned that we should make an appointment with her doctor about her misplacing things. Thankfully, she agreed. We saw her doctor in July and he scheduled the CAT-Scan and EEG.

I began noticing she was having trouble with words. She wasn't really struggling to remember words. Not yet. She would be speaking and use the wrong word in a sentence. A word that had nothing to do with the word she meant to use. Her brain seemed to have sent a signal for this random word. One little word out of place. She never realized this was happening and I never pointed it out. I couldn't help but worry more.

She started having trouble with time shortly after that first doctor appointment. Not with telling time so much. More like the concept of time. She would ask me the time and I'd tell her it was 1 PM. She'd ask when the grandkids got out of school and I'd say 3 PM. Then she would ask if she should leave to go get them. I'd tell her there was plenty of time and I'd let her know when she needed to leave. Ten minutes later, she'd ask again. And then again. I always tried to answer her like it was the first time she asked. It's so important to not point out their lapse in memory. The only thing this would gain is frustrating her. The last thing I wanted was for her to be worrying about anything.

The problem she had with time progressed beyond the hours of a day. She started having trouble understand the amount of time between days in a week. Even the year became an issue. She wanted to start writing appointments and school events on a calendar. Unfortunately, she kept trying to write them on a 2017 calendar. No amount of explaining could get her to understand the year was 2016. So, I would let her write the appointments and events on the 2017 calendar.

This concept of time issue seemed to be the most affected part of her memory. It's what worried me the most. Her long-term memory was as clear as ever at this point. I had to leave for a 1 PM appointment one day. I picked up Jade at the high school after my appointment. I got home around 3:30 PM. Our oldest granddaughter Sage told me her grandmother had gone out and sat on the porch as soon as I had left. She said she asked her what she was doing on the porch. Marsha told her she was waiting for the school bus to drop Harmonie, our youngest granddaughter, off. She had sat on the porch for two and a half hours wondering where the bus was.

The next new occurrence happened in October 2016. I decided we would drive the granddaughters to New York City for their fall break from school. Marsha and I loved *The Phantom of the Opera*, especially on Broadway. We had seen it five times over the years. I wanted the two of us to share this experience with the granddaughters. More importantly, I wanted to do this while Marsha could still enjoy this special moment with the girls. And them with her.

The trip is about an eleven-hour drive under normal circumstances. It's never normal when we travel. We must make stops every hour because of my bad legs and blood clot issues. Typically, I'd drive a couple hours and then she would drive a couple hours until reaching our destination. Not this trip. She was out of sorts the whole time she was in the car. She had trouble remembering where we were at or what state we were in. She couldn't understand the directions I printed out from MapQuest. I tried to let her drive some so I could nap. I told her to stay on this specific highway for the next three hours. This didn't work out very long. Her having no concept of time didn't help. Every exit we hit she would wake me up to ask if she should take it. I ended up driving most of the trip.

She didn't travel as a passenger much better. The small confines of the van made her irritable. Very irritable. Our stops to stretch legs and use the bathroom helped but not enough. Toward the end of the trip, she would be angry. I couldn't help but be reminded of the last time we drove Mamaw to Mom's house on the lake. The similarities of these two trips terrified me.

Chapter 15
Two Become One

Marsha and I first met in December 1990 at *Fit for Life*, a local gym. I had seen her before, kind of admiring her beauty from a distance, but we had never spoken. I was recently divorced and had my three kids, Amber, Bobby, and Robby for the weekend. I had brought the kids with me to the gym so they could swim while I lifted weights. This beautiful woman I had admired from afar approached me that day. I had no idea what she wanted but I was nervous. She said, "Excuse me, are those your kids in the pool area?"

Uh oh… I thought. *I wonder what they had done.*

"You might want to go check on them," she politely informed me.

Oh boy, this was not the conversation I expected to be having with her.

I headed toward the pool room expecting the worse. I was overcome with guilt as soon as I saw my kids. They weren't hanging from the ceiling or wrestling around in the pool. They weren't in a time-out with a staff member waiting to scold me. Nope. My kids were sound asleep on the pool deck. They looked like they had used their last bit of energy to climb out of the pool before conking out from exhaustion. I felt horrible for not checking on them sooner. I gently woke each of them and coaxed them toward the locker rooms. I thanked Marsha on the way out the door. I had no idea who she was when I left. I was too ashamed to ask.

I had met Dave Roberts years earlier at the gym. We were on similar workout schedules so I saw him there most of the time. A friendship quickly developed as we got to know each other. Lucky for me, Dave worked with Marsha at Crane. He approached me one day and pointed toward Marsha. She was riding a stationary bike across from where we were. He asked me if I'd like to meet her. Obviously, I told him, "Absolutely." I then mentioned that I didn't think she would be interested in meeting me. He laughed and bet me a case of Coke she would. He took me over to the bikes and introduced us. I thanked her again for telling me about my sleeping kids and apologized for letting it happen. We visited for a bit before going our separate ways.

She was at the gym every time I went. I always went to the bikes to visit with her as soon as I saw she was on one. We both liked to sit in the sauna after our workouts. I tried to finish my workout at the same time as her so we'd be in the sauna together. I sound like a pervert but we had some good visits in the sauna. We learned a lot about each other during those visits.

She was a government employee and worked at Crane Army Ammunition. Crane made the smart boards for most missiles and many of the bombs the military used. They also made most of the batteries for the military. She was a Department of Defense employee but worked as a budget analyst for the Army. She had two daughters, Natalie and Bambie. Natalie was on her own then and worked at Indiana University. Bambie was fourteen and still lived at home. She had been separated from her husband for quite some time. They couldn't finalize the divorce because of difficulties in splitting their assets. We went on our first date in January of 1991.

We quickly connected and knew there was no one else for us. We were meant to be together. Three months later, she sold her house. I was managing two hotels at the time, the Stonehenge Lodge here in Bedford and the Howard Johnson in Clarksville, Indiana. I was living out of both. She moved in with me at Stonehenge in May. I got full custody of my three kids around the end of June. Marsha and I bought a huge four-bedroom house on seventeen acres. We lived in an apartment in the hotel for a month before moving into our house in July. Her divorce was finalized around the same time.

I proposed to her in the fall. We didn't set a date. We just made it official that we were going to get hitched. That winter, we decided to fly to Las Vegas with my mother and Bob Reed to get married. We both agreed we didn't want a large wedding since we had both been married before. Vegas was the perfect choice. Mom and Bob paid for our trip. We arrived in Vegas the last week of March with no date set. Neither of us had ever been there before so I spent most of the first few days gambling. Marsha and Mom did a lot of shopping. I was playing craps with Bob on the third day when Marsha brought up the wedding. I told her I didn't care where we got married so she could choose whatever location made her happy. Big mistake. A little while later, she came back down to the casino with a wide grin on her face. She proceeded to try and convince me to have a medieval wedding on horseback. Not only that, she wanted to get married on April 1. An April Fool's Day wedding. Fortunately for me, she was joking. She then asked me to come up to the room and help her decide on a location.

Weddings are a big deal in Vegas. The yellow pages were loaded with different venues. There were tons of advertisements for every theme imaginable. Things like gothic, on horseback, and even drive-thru weddings where you didn't have to leave your car. We could have had an Elvis impersonator conduct the ceremony or dozens of other celebrity impersonators. I'm old fashion and believe in traditional things. Weddings should be in a church with a preacher not on horseback in a fake Nottingham Woods. We decided on the Little Church of the West. It was a small church with a history of celebrity weddings to add a little uniqueness to our wedding.

The chapel was the first chapel in Las Vegas built as a wedding chapel and not a church. The wedding scene of Elvis Presley and Ann Margaret in the movie *Viva Las Vegas* was shot inside the chapel. Both Judy Garland and Mickey Rooney each held one of their many weddings in the chapel. Cindy Crawford, Richard Gere, and Dudley Moore also married spouses in this little church. To me, it will forever be known as the place where Bob and Marsha Kern shared their wedding vows on March 30, 1992. We both agreed it would make for a great story to be married in this historical little chapel.[i]

All four of us drove to the Little Church of the West to make the wedding arrangements. The church was owned by the Hacienda Casino back then. It sat right outside the hotel and casino entrance. It's called Little Church of the West for a reason. It was very small. Very small. We parked out front and entered the church into a tiny foyer. Once inside, I could see a double door that led inside the actual sanctuary. There wasn't a wedding going on so the doors were open. The chapel was more like a replica of a church. Something little girls might have built in their backyards. An aisle ran down the center of the sanctuary to the small pulpit. Five rows of pews were running along both sides of the aisle. Each pew was tiny as well, no more than a two-seater.

We were greeted by a kind lady who took us into an office located to the side of the foyer. The office had a desk and a single board on the wall. The board displayed the various wedding packages they offered. I splurged for my bride-to-be and bought the premium package – Wedding Package A. This covered the cost of the wedding, a video recording of it, a fresh flower bouquet, and a complimentary bottle of champagne. Nothing but the best for my soon-to-be wife. We selected our time for the afternoon of March 30. I then had to pay upfront for the wedding, which was nonrefundable. This made sense, considering where we were. I'm sure many minds get changed when the alcohol wears off.

That was easy enough. Next, we had to get a marriage license. We left the church and headed to the county courthouse. We entered the courthouse without issue and headed for the elevators. Once we arrived on the proper floor, we had to find the county clerk's office that issued wedding licenses. It turned out to be easy to find. They had a metal detector and a couple county police officers outside the door. This was March 1992, a decade before 9/11. We couldn't believe it. Of all the places in Vegas you could come and go without issue, you had to walk through a metal detector to get a marriage license. All four of us laughed about this for years.

The afternoon of March 30 rolled around and Bob and I put on our business suits. I wore one of my black suits with a red tie to look a little more formal. Marsha wore a beautiful ivory dress. She looked like an angel to me. She still does. Bob got the hotel to provide a limousine so we rode in style to the chapel. I could tell Marsha was a little nervous on the ride over there. I could also tell it was the ceremony, not me, that had her this way. She was beaming the whole ride.

We arrived a few minutes early and were ushered directly into the sanctuary. The double doors were closed behind us and the ceremony began. The ceremony was a quick one but still followed the traditional procedures. Our vows were the standard ones, straight from the Bible. Bob stood next to me as my best man and mom by Marsha as her Maid of Honor. Vows were said, rings exchanged, and I kissed my beautiful bride. The whole thing was over before I knew it. Wedding music was played as we all headed toward the now open door. I heard a bell ring as we exited the sanctuary. Either an angel had just gotten their wings or the ceremony was officially concluded. We were all taken to the side of the foyer to sign the wedding certificates. The preacher had already signed in his spots. I watched as another wedding party entered the sanctuary while we were signing. I found myself laughing out loud when the chapel doors closed for their wedding. The staff member with us quickly hushed me. On the back of the now closed door was a sign that read, *Quiet Please. Wedding in Progress.* Talk about efficient. These people didn't waste any time cranking out newlyweds. Twenty-five years later and we couldn't be happier. Even with this dreadful disease.

I have been blessed with a wonderful life with this woman. We have raised five kids together. When our youngest three were in high school, we were further blessed to have our granddaughters, Sage and Jade become part of our life. We ended up adopting them. Events occurred which brought the girl's little sister, Harmonie, into our lives. We haven't been able to experience life as empty-nesters but you won't hear me complain. Neither of us can imagine life without them in it.

Chapter 16
God's Hand

Life goes on whether we want it to or not. Our children and grandchildren enter this world as babies depending on us to care and provide for them. They crawl, and in a blink of an eye, they're walking. We tell ourselves they're growing up too fast. But they keep growing. They become more and more independent and less and less dependent on us. Yet, we do nothing. We think it's out of our control.

Kids are supposed to grow into adults. They are supposed to start their own families and have their own lives. We work hard and raise them the best we can for this moment. Then we look back and wonder where the time went. How did they grow up so fast? It seems like it was only the other day we cradled them in our arms. Where did the time go? Guilt creeps in as we wish we had spent more time with them when they were young. It's too late now. They're gone. Off raising their own families.

I got out of the Army in 1988 and went straight into running the Stonehenge Lodge. A year later, I started running a second hotel, the Howard Johnson Hotel, an hour away. I was used to working long hours in the Army so it seemed natural to continue working seventy and eighty hour weeks. I always tried to take Sundays off for my family. I was an extreme workaholic the rest of the week. I also lifted weights like a madman two or three days a week. I lifted like I worked until my muscles were completely exhausted. This helped me sleep better when I got home. I got out of the business in 2001 but found myself back in it in 2005. I slipped right back into that workaholic mode and was killing myself. I left this hotel in February 2008.

In July 2008, I was volunteering at a church camp when my body succumbed to eight years in the infantry and sixteen years of hotel management. I went to bed the first night of camp with every muscle in my body screaming in pain and completely exhausted. I woke up the next morning with no improvement. I worked all day and barely made it to my dorm before falling to sleep. Same thing the next morning. No change. I hurt all over and was exhausted. Something was seriously wrong. I finished the final two days of camp certain I was on death's bed. That Monday, I went to my doctor. He sent me to a rheumatologist that specializes in auto-immune diseases. I was diagnosed with chronic pain, chronic fatigue, fibromyalgia, sleep apnea, severe restless leg syndrome, depression, and neuropathy. Plus, my history of blood clots. He sent me to the Mayo Clinic in December 2009 where I underwent a week of all day tests. The clinic confirmed my rheumatologist's diagnoses. The theory was my body had been pushed to its limits for so many years suppressing my immune system. I must have caught a virus that created the perfect storm in me, spiraling into all these different ailments. By the time the virus had worked its way out of my system, the damage was done.

Since July 2008, I live every day in severe pain. Pain and exhaustion that is intensified by any physical activities. I can't take the recommended treatments of anti-inflammatories like Ibuprofen because of the blood thinners I am on. It took a few years but I got the right combination of medicines to get me through the day. My life is built around routines and if I overdo it, I know there will be a price to pay. I'll end the pity party here.

I believe my health issues were God's way of getting my attention. I was a workaholic my whole life. That's how I was wired. The only way for this to change was to take away my ability to work for good. And He did. Three months later, we welcomed Harmonie into our home and got permanent guardianship of her. Sage was ten years old and Jade had recently turned nine years old when their little sister joined us that October. Harmonie turned three years old the next month. Our three granddaughters needed a stay-at-home parent and circumstances allowed me to be there for them.

I took care of the kids for the next five years while Marsha worked. I got Sage and Jade off to school and Harmonie to preschool at Crossroads Church. I did light chores around the house each day to keep it clean. My days were regimented because of my health so I never planned anything beyond the current day. I'd go to the store every day to shop for that evening's supper. The kids would be famished by the end of the school day. They ate lunch so early I had to have their supper ready when they got home. I'd be exhausted when they got home. My last chore was to wash the dishes. I could hit my recliner for the rest of the night when this was done. It was homework time for the girls once they had eaten. They would climb up in the recliner with me if they needed help and we'd work on it together. They would bring me their work to check before being able to go outside and play. Every night, one of them had dance lessons except Wednesday, which was church night. Bedtime came around at 8 PM for the kids. Marsha and I weren't up much longer. I was so tired and in so much pain by this time I would fall asleep instantly. Life was great. It took some serious health issues to get me here, but my feet were, at long last, on the right path.

I was living my life one day at a time. All my energy and focus was on my family. This meant I got to spend valuable time with my granddaughters as they grew up. I didn't miss any life events with them. No regrets or wishing they weren't growing up so fast. I could be present for everything. During summer breaks, I got to spend every waking moment with the girls. We took trips to state parks, museums, the library, or spent the day swimming in our pool. I was home when Marsha got off work. I was with her all day on her days off. Life had put me in a place where I no longer had to concern myself with anything. I was truly living completely in the moment.

The next few years, Marsha's work got more and more demanding for her. She has gotten horrible migraines her whole life. It got so bad that she was coming home with them several days a week. Other nights she came home and simply broke down and cried. It broke my heart. I'd had enough of seeing the toll her work was having on her. I decided it was time to talk to her about retiring. The work was killing her and I was starting to need some help at home. It was beginning to get harder for me to get through the day. She filed her retirement papers for the end of the year. After thirty-nine years as a government employee, she retired December 31, 2112.

Her retirement was all that was missing to complete the perfect life for me. I'm an early riser so I got the kids to and from school. She took over preparing dinner and driving them to their evening activities. It's only the two of us during the day. We were homebodies so our focus was on the girls and each other. She occasionally got together for lunch with friends. Otherwise, our activities centered on the five of us. And, of course, church every week.

I believe this had God's hand in it. I got sick and couldn't work anymore around the same time we needed to care for another grandchild. A toddler still in diapers and needs lots of love and attention. Above all, when they're old enough to know they aren't with their mommy anymore. We had three granddaughters that were the center of our universe. These kids needed someone fully involved in their lives. They had me for four years and now both of us were home for them. I believe with all my heart that everything happened to get me in this place. A place where I love my life and cherish every day, living each day as it comes.

I had witnessed the loss of Marsha's father to Alzheimer's and how it affected us. Then Mamaw falling at my house while visiting for the day. This blessed me with a chance to be with her every day of her final years. I witnessed up-close how dementia stripped Mamaw of everything before taking her life. I made sure she was never alone, no matter what.

My health deteriorated as Marsha's work stress became too much. She retired and enjoyed five wonderful years with me and the girls. More importantly, the girls and I got to spend this time with her. Living each day as it comes and enjoying it to the fullest. We are all truly blessed.

I have always believed everything happens for a reason. I never look back with regret. I believe we all go through trials and tribulations, good choices and bad choices, all to get where we are at. Besides, looking back only causes you to miss something in the now. How can I regret a bad first marriage that produced me three great kids? How can I complain about living every day with pain and fatigue? I can't when I get to spend every day with my lovely wife and precious granddaughters.

Everything in life has prepared me to deal with my wife's dementia. I truly believe this. It allows me to spend real quality time with her every day. I can devote myself completely to her and the kids. I'm right there next to her to keep her calm when she forgets things. I can ensure her happiness every day as we approach each one together. March 30, 2017, is our Silver Anniversary. Twenty-five years with this wonderful woman. God willing, I'll get to spend many more years with her. I'm grateful for each day.

Chapter 17
Our New Normal

My wonderful life continues even after the diagnoses. I continue to live each day as it comes. My only goal each day is to make sure my wife is happy. Obviously, I've adjusted my own routines around her condition. I'll continue adjusting as her dementia worsens. I'll be honest, it's not easy. It's hard some days to keep from thinking about her diagnoses. Thinking about it chokes me up. The last thing I want is for her to see me crying. This only upsets her and gets her thinking about the future.

Her doctor never confirmed the diagnoses of Alzheimer's so she remains very adamant that she doesn't have it. She knew her CAT-Scan showed atrophy on the left and right sides of her frontal lobe. She is aware that this is the cause of her dementia. Her doctor told her the two medicines she is on can improve her dementia. He asks us at every visit if we could see any improvement in her symptoms. She seemed happier. She always told him she thought she was better. I never contradicted her. I didn't have the heart to take away her hope. I would tell him she still had no concept of time and trouble finding words. She could read a clock but couldn't grasp the value of it. I did notice the medicine was making her less stressed.

Her doctor suggested she do activities that challenge her brain. He explained that she might be able to retrain her brain. The objective was for other parts of her brain to resume the functions that the atrophied parts used to do. I don't believe this is true. Everything I've read about dementia indicated there was no cure. At least not for dementia caused by Alzheimer's and strokes. Even the medicines prescribed state they will not cure or heal the dementia. The hope is the medication will slow down the progression.

I got her Sudoku books but even the easy ones were too hard for her. I also got Search-A-Word puzzles and she does well with them. She loves doing puzzles so we bought a five-hundred-piece puzzle to start with. Our son Rob usually visits on his days off from work. The two of them have a wonderful time working together on these puzzles. They're working on one-thousand-piece puzzles now. I've tried to get her to read. She enjoyed reading the first draft of my autobiography before I published it in February 2015 because it made her laugh. She decided she wanted to read the published version recently. It was obvious right away that this was tough for her. She simply couldn't stick to it very long. I don't know if it was a concentration issue or a problem recognizing words. I didn't ask about it. Both are issues that would draw her attention to the dementia. Nothing good would come from that. I focus on the things she can do. The things that will make her feel good when she completes them.

She went through a brief period where she would get up early. A thought would enter her head and she couldn't stop thinking about it. She still can't sleep in on days she has an appointment. It doesn't matter how late in the day her appointment might be. This is because of her trouble with time. She would worry herself sick that she'd be late for it. I'd coax her back to bed while reassuring her we had plenty of time. Next thing I'd know, I would hear the hot water tank kick on. She was up and in the shower. This was okay. It meant she'd be up with me longer while we waited for her appointment.

We like spending time together on our reclining love seat. Watching the TV shows we recorded from the night before is quality time for us. Oddly, the Alzheimer's commercials don't bother her. I cringe every time they come on but she never reacts to them. Sometimes, she will start crying for no reason or from something she heard on the TV. I'll ask her what's wrong right away when she cries. She'll tell me she doesn't want to die. It breaks my heart when this happens. I do my best to comfort her while I fight back my own tears. I'll hold her in my arms and tell her she is going to be fine and we'll get through this together. These moments are extremely hard for me. I can't imagine life without her. I try to block these thoughts out but when she has these breakdowns they go straight to my heart.

She has stopped using the wrong words in her sentences. Instead, she began having trouble finding the right word. She would be speaking and her brain seems to get stuck and she can't find the word. I will try to help her as soon as I hear her struggling. Sometimes, I will be clueless about the word she is searching for. I will say something light-hearted before she can get frustrated. I say something like, "I'm sorry sweetheart, but I'm going to need a little more information to help you here." Or, "I'm sorry babe, but something's blocking your brainwaves and I can't read your mind." Most of the time, I know what word she needed as soon as she paused. When you've been together like we have, you become of one mind. You know each other so well you can complete each other's thoughts.

She has started sleeping longer than she used to. She rarely gets up before 9 AM and some days, she will sleep until 11 AM. I check on her frequently while she's sleeping. I don't know why, but I always check to make sure she is still breathing. There are days when she'll get up and stay in her pajamas all day. She won't shower and get dressed until it's time to pick the kids up at 3 PM. This doesn't bother me since she's comfortable and happy. It only concerns me because I remember Mom saying Mamaw started staying in her pajamas as she got worse. I try not to think about this as difficult as it is.

I've started missing a lot of church services on Sunday. This is something that really bothers me. I don't feel right missing church, I never have. It's not that I've lost my faith, it remains as strong as ever. It's just that I feel bad leaving her in bed asleep when I go. It terrifies me she'll wake up and panic if she can't find me. The few times I have gone without her, I sit in the pew fighting back tears. Everything reminds me of her dementia. The songs we sing, the preacher's message, everything pulls at my heart. My eyes start swelling up and I end up fighting to control my emotions. It doesn't help having an empty spot next to me where she usually sits. I sometimes see my preacher up on the stage wiping his eyes during the worship songs when he sees me struggling. I've committed to getting the whole family back into our church routines. We need that fellowship and additional praying now more than ever.

After some time, we started letting people know about her diagnoses. Since then, I've noticed most of our friends have shied away from us. Particularly, hers. Her phone used to go off all day long with phone calls and text messages. Not so much anymore. Sometimes, she'll comment she's surprised she hasn't gotten any visitors at our home since this. Other times, she'll remark that she hasn't heard from this person or that person in a while. Dementia isn't contagious. I understand people's reluctance to be around. The word Alzheimer's and dementia conjure unpleasant images. I don't understand why anyone would have an issue seeing her in the initial stages. She still recognizes people. She is still the same loving, caring person everyone knows. There's no reason for anyone to cut off contact with someone because of dementia. If anything, this is when they need interaction with loved ones and friends the most. They still retain most of the faculties but they're scared about the memories they are losing. Having normal conversations with people she knows would be so beneficial. It would certainly help to make her feel normal.

She still gets out occasionally. She'll have breakfast or lunch with one of her longtime friends. Our church's helping hands committee recently encouraged her to come to their monthly dinner. She was a member of the committee for years. She was ready to come home after an hour or two away. This is a typical tendency for people with dementia. They get to a point where an unfamiliar environment begins making them nervous. She'll begin feeling this way and tell her friends she needs to get home.

I Know Marsha feels my absence from her side. I am always right there with her and she finds comfort in this. I am her anchor. I suspect knowing I'm near helps keep her calm, when her memory falters or she gets confused. When I leave the room for very long she'll always come find me. Sometimes, she'll follow me around the house so she can keep me in her sight. It's no problem for me. If it makes her feel better keeping me in sight and staying by my side, that's fine by me. This gives me more time with her.

I try to write books. It's a little more difficult but I adjust to the challenges. I am currently working on books four, five, and six in my 'We Were Soldiers Too' series. This project continues to be very important to me, but not as important as my wife. I still plan on finishing at least the fifteen books in my business plan for the series. It's a little more difficult to get in a groove writing with her dementia. I have trouble some days finding the time for the phone interviews with the veterans I feature in each book. I must be more patient now when writing. I get interrupted a lot. She has lots of questions throughout the day. Sometimes, she just likes to talk so I stop writing and listen to what she says. She struggles with electronics and I stop and help her with this. Other times, I see her sitting somewhere by herself and I can feel myself getting emotional.

I stop writing and go sit next to her, placing my arm around her. Moments like this are worth more to me than any book I might write.

My new role requires me to provide comic relief throughout each day. No, I don't sit around all day cracking jokes to make her laugh. I do try to keep the mood light as much as I can. I have a good sense of humor, which helps. I'll tease her about misspoken words or lost items. She tends to change her clothes quite often and I'll tease her about this. Nothing mean-spirited. Only little, light-hearted jabs to make her laugh. She likes gestures of affection. Little reminders that she is loved. I make sure to hug and kiss her as frequently as possible throughout the day. I try to tell her I love her all day long. She responds to this with pure joy. You haven't lived until you've seen someone completely light up from your gestures of love. Such a small task for me with such a huge reward. I am so blessed.

It's not all rainbows and unicorns. I have days where it's hard for me to be patient all day long. I unintentionally get snippy with her. I apologize when this happens, at once. It's not her fault she forgets things. I have weak moments when I think about losing her and it tears me up. I'm not always able to reign my emotions in and control them. Sometimes, it all catches up to me and it's too much. I've had a few episodes at 5 AM in the shower where my bodies awake but my mind still has one foot in dreamland. My mind will latch to the thought of a life without her. Before I know what's happened, I'll be standing in the shower crying like a baby. Thank God, these episodes tend to occur when I am alone. If she were to catch me in one of these weaker moments, it would crush her. For her, and her happiness, I fight to keep these feelings buried in the deep recesses of my mind so I can focus on her.

Chapter 18
Closing

I continue to live life day-by-day. This allows me to enjoy every precious one of them with my beautiful wife. I have no idea what the future holds for us. I refuse to look that far ahead. I am perfectly content to be living in the moment. I know firsthand what to expect from her dementia as it continues with its deathly grip on her. Dwelling on it will only keep me from enjoying the time we have left together. I could die tomorrow, for all I know. Thinking about our mortality affects our ability to enjoy a higher quality of life while we're living. I will not let the things out of my control affect the things I can control.

I pray that a cure for this awful disease is found before it's too late for her. I pray that God will cure her so that she doesn't have to leave me this way. I pray that He will let me take her illness upon myself and to let her live her days out without this affliction. I would take this illness from her in a heartbeat if He would let me. If it's not in His will to do any of this, I pray He will free her mind from worry and will allow her to spend her final time on this earth happy. I leave it all in God's merciful hands so I can give her the attention and devotion she needs.

I see no other way to look at this. Any attention or energy I place elsewhere only takes away from what's important - my time with her. I have no idea how much time I will have with her. This is one of the great dilemmas of this disease. Dementia has no timetable. There's no specific progression of the symptoms to gauge what stage of the disease someone is in. The consensus would be eight to ten years from detection of the initial stages. Some people have lived twenty years from the first detection. Then with others, the progression happens quickly over a few years from the first symptoms of the disease. It doesn't help that symptoms tend to go unnoticed the first few years. The signs may seem insignificant, be ignored as part of aging, or be hidden by the inflicted person. This proves it is simply impossible to have any viable way to provide a timetable for this. I refuse to worry about any of this, but I do pray it's twenty.

What we do know is, it's deadly. It's one of the worse diseases on earth. Why? It is pure torture to watch a loved one slowly lose everything and know there is nothing that can be done for them. Their entire identity is stripped from them. We are forced to stand by as they lose their short-term memory. Then they start forgetting the names of friends and family. They end up all alone with no idea who or what is around them. Everything is an unknown to them. This certainly must be a terrifying way to go through each day. They're forced to go through this deterioration of their memories, isolated from humanity. They roam the corridors of life feeling alone and lost. And we can only watch. Then the disease strips them of their dignity by destroying the brain's ability to control their body's functions. They forget how to walk and end up locked in a foreign world stuck in bed or a chair, the ultimate feeling of loneliness. The disease isn't done yet. It has more sinister work to do by stealing the memories required for eating. We are forced to be helpless observers as our loved ones slide through these horrible stages. Stripped of everything yet, the disease still isn't done. We are forced to silently witness their bodies deteriorate to nothing before they are released to be with our Lord and Savior.

This is too much for me to dwell on. My heart was broken when I lost my mamaw. I still feel that sorrow. I'm not sure I can survive the heartbreak of losing my dear, sweet wife. I don't know how I will be able to go on. I have faith that God will be there.

For now, I only want to enjoy what we have. The life we've built together. Our children and grandchildren. And each day that I am blessed to be with this wonderful woman.

She will never walk alone.

Edited by Toni Michelle
http://www.polishedpagesediting.com/

www.bobkernauthor.com

They Walk Alone/ Bob Kern. -- 1st edition.

"I Can Do All Things Through Christ Who Strengthens Me" — Philippians 4:13

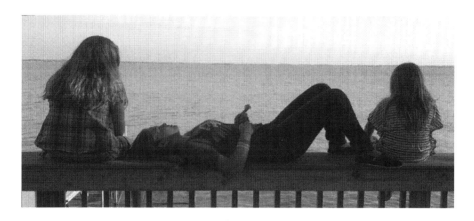

Resides in Bedford, Indiana with his wife Marsha and their three granddaughters; Sage, Jade, and Harmonie. Father to five children; Natalie, Bambie, Amber, Bob Jr, and Rob. Additional grandchildren: Daven, Haeven, Makarah, Blake, and Kerrigan.

Served in the United States Army from November 1980 to March 1988. Service awards: Expert Infantry Badge, Army Commendation Medal (2), Army Achievement Medal (8), NCO Development Ribbon (2), Good Conduct Medal (2), Overseas Ribbon, Worked as general manager of two full service hotels from 1988 to 2001. During this period, he founded and served ten years on the Lawrence County tourism commission.

https://www.bobkernauthor.com/

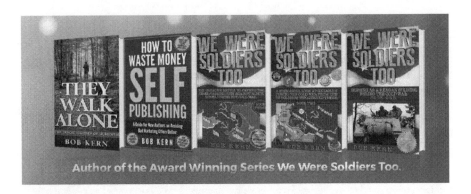

Author of the Award Winning Series We Were Soldiers Too.

Bob is the author of the award-winning series *We Were Soldiers Too*. Due to the overwhelming support and response from other Cold War Veterans, there are plans for twelve books in the series. We Were Soldiers Too is a Cold War documentary series that tells the history of the Cold War from the perspective of the veterans who served during this critical time in history.

The first book in the series was about his time in the military and was a finalist for Nonfiction Autobiography of the Year in 2015 with the Independent Authors Network.

Book Two is on serving in Germany during the Cold War. It has won awards in numerous contests in the nonfiction category. The book received a Bronze Medal from the Nonfiction Authors Association. It was a Finalist for eBook of the Year with Next Generation Indie Book Awards, Finalist for Military History Book of the Year with National Indie Excellence Awards, Finalist for Nonfiction History with Independent Authors Network. Most recently, it won third place and the Bronze Medal from the prestigious Dan Poynter's Global eBook Awards in the Nonfiction-Military category and Honorable Mention in Nonfiction- History with one of the largest book contests, the Reader's Favorite Book Awards. It was also awarded a 5-star review for Readers Favorite Books.

Book three, serving in Korea during the Cold War, was named Nonfiction Military History BOOK OF THE YEAR.

Book four, Defending the Iron Curtain will be released June 1, 2017

Book five, Inside the DMZ- The Most Fortified Border in the World is scheduled to be released in late July 2017

He is currently working on book six, 1983- On the Verge of Nuclear War and book seven, Ghost Walkers in the DMZ. These two are expected to be released towards the end of 2017.

In January 2017, he released, How to Waste Money Self-Publishing" a short book for new authors. The book covers many of the pitfalls and scams to avoid when trying to market books. It also shares information and tips on publishing your own book.

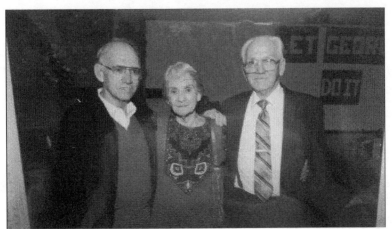

The above photo was taken at Marta's house in 1999. This was Mamaw's last visit there as mentioned in introduction. The dashing young man on the right is her baby brother, my Uncle Phil Solomon. The handsome young man on the right is her brother, my Uncle George Solomon. The "Let George Do It" in the background was the motto for Uncle George's one-man (and daughter Marta) construction company.

To my beautiful wife, Marsha, who is more than my better half. She completes me. Together we are one. The biggest blessing God ever gave me was you sweetheart. Words can't do justice to the way I feel about you. My love for you will never end.

For my beloved mother, Sheryl, and the amazing job you did raising us five kids by yourself. The strength, character, and integrity she always maintained and the positive example she set for us, still inspires me. We had no money but were never poor. And to my siblings Scott Kern, Laura Reddick, James Kern, and Amy Kern-Smith. Words cannot describe the honor I feel in being your big brother

In loving memory of my dear, sweet Mamaw. She continues to make the world a better place through the lives of all the people she touched during her time with us. Thank you Lord for blessing me and making her my Mamaw.

In loving memory of David and Dottie Lyons who went to the Lord to soon. You gave me the greatest gift ever when you gave your blessings for me to marry your daughter.

---

[i] https://littlechurchlv.com/chapel-tour/, February 1, 2017

Made in the USA
Columbia, SC
07 January 2024

29284182R10078